FIRE UP
Your Metabolism

---

9 PROVEN PRINCIPLES FOR BURNING FAT AND LOSING WEIGHT FOREVER

Lyssie Lakatos, R.D., and
Tammy Lakatos Shames, R.D.

A FIRESIDE BOOK
Published by Simon & Schuster
New York   London   Toronto   Sydney

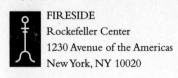

FIRESIDE
Rockefeller Center
1230 Avenue of the Americas
New York, NY 10020

FIRESIDE and colophon are registered trademarks
of Simon & Schuster, Inc.

For information regarding special discounts for bulk purchases, please contact Simon
& Schuster Special Sales: 1-800-456-6798 or business@simonandschuster.com

Designed by Kris Tobiassen

Manufactured in the United States of America

10 9 8 7 6 5 4 3 2 1

Library of Congress Cataloging-in-Publication Data

Lakatos, Lyssie.
    Fire up your metabolism: 9 proven principles for burning fat and losing weight
forever/Lyssie Lakatos and Tammy Lakatos Shames.
        p.   cm.
    Includes index.
    1. Weight loss.   2. Metabolism—Regulation.
I. Shames, Tammy Lakatos.   II. Title.

RM222.2.L285 2004
613.2'5—dc22   2003 061710
ISBN 0-7432-4548-2

To Scott, Mom, and Dad

ACKNOWLEDGMENTS

First and foremost we would like to thank our clients who have inspired us to write this book. Their success and encouragement helped us to realize that we could make it possible for others to fire up their metabolism.

We would like to thank our amazing literary agent, Laura Dail, of Laura Dail Literary Agency, for making this book a reality. Thank you so much for believing in us and for working your magic.

Our warmest thanks to everyone at Simon and Schuster, especially our wonderful editor, Doris Cooper, whose incredible vision helped mold this book. We feel so lucky to have had the opportunity to work with you and we truly couldn't ask for a more insightful editor. You are the best. Thank you.

Many thanks to our copy editor, Cynthia Merman, for being so thoughtful and thorough.

We'd like to thank Heidi Mochari and Doug Kalman who were always so willing to share their plethora of nutritional knowledge.

On a personal note, thanks to our incredible friends and family for always being there for us.

Thanks to Mom and Dad, for your love and support in everything we do—without you both, we would never be where we are today.

And to Tammy's husband, Scott, words cannot express enough thanks for your constant love, understanding, and patience, and for putting up with the long hours and late nights—not to mention dealing with Tammy when it was her turn be the "guinea pig" in our trials. Thank you for your motivation and encouragement.

CONTENTS

INTRODUCTION

Dieters today are frustrated and discouraged. Their strict eating plans are carried out in vain and their trips to the gym don't pay off. If they do see some success, their results quickly vanish as soon as they veer— even slightly—from regimented diet and exercise programs.

Why?

Many people don't burn calories *efficiently,* and they store food as fat rather than burning it up for energy.

Frustrated dieters simply need to *fire up* their metabolism.

So now you may be saying, "What exactly is metabolism and how can I fire up mine?"

Simply, metabolism is the way your body uses calories from the food you eat. The speed at which it does so is called your metabolic rate. Everyone who likes to eat wants to have a speedy metabolism so that they can burn food for energy without storing it as fat, which is what happens when the metabolic rate is slow. Unfortunately, the body's natural tendency is to slow the metabolism and store food as fat, causing weight gain.

Yet no one is doomed by these factors.

People who have a slow metabolism often blame their weight gain on their genes. Or their age. Or their inactive jobs. They don't realize that they can burn more calories by making relatively *small* changes in their diet and lifestyle.

★ ★ ★

It's probably not news to you that what you eat and how you live affect your weight. Despite this, desperate dieters want a quick fix, and they jump to try the newest fad diet, such as the Atkins Diet, Sugar Busters!, and The Zone in hopes of seeing quick weight loss.

These diets can cause an initial quick weight loss, but when they do this, they do something else, too: They actually *slow* the metabolism. And that *hinders* long-term weight loss.

We are all too familiar with the embarrassed dieter who rebounds to a higher weight after each round of dieting.

When weight fluctuates in this manner, not only is body composition altered, but so is metabolism. *You see, chronic dieting transforms metabolism to favor weight gain.*

Why?

Because each time you lose weight, you also lose lean muscle tissue. Lean muscle tissue needs calories simply to exist. So the more times you gain and lose weight, the more lean muscle tissue you lose, and the fewer calories your body burns.

When you fire up your metabolism, you are not going on a diet. So there's no such thing as "cheating." Yes, you will make some changes to what you eat, but more than anything you are changing the way your body uses food.

On the Fire Up Your Metabolism plan, you will try to apply as many metabolism-revving tips to your life as possible—and you *will see results*. This plan will become your nutrition and fitness bible, your way of life, a lifestyle that keeps your metabolism on high. You can have that cookie. Take a bunch of french fries. Enjoy a slice of pizza. Relish your favorite foods. You can't have a lot every day, but you don't have to swear off the foods you love to fire up your metabolism.

After reading our book and following our tips, you will lose weight and keep it off—without feeling deprived. Whether you are a man in your mid-twenties trying to stave off a gut, or a menopausal woman, our strategies combined with the nutrition principles we explain in plain language will help anyone who has struggled to achieve a thinner body. Weakness and lethargy will be feelings of the past.

This is not a fad diet book. It's a plan that adheres to the recommendations of the American Heart Association and the American Dietetic Association. The plan is rooted in nine principles that will teach you how to speed up your metabolic rate:

1. Never skip meals.
2. Eat at the right times.
3. Choose a diet rich in the best carbohydrates.
4. Appropriately time intake of lean proteins.
5. Drink appropriate amounts of certain beverages at specific times.
6. Eat a diet low in "bad" fat.
7. Get enough sleep every night.
8. Find surprising ways to stay active.
9. Incorporate muscle strengthening in your exercise routines.

You may have heard these suggestions before yet not fully understood how to incorporate them into your eating and lifestyle habits. Or, like many of our clients, you may be suspicious of anything that promises weight loss. We are, too. Not only will we tell you what to do, but we will explain *why* it's important for revving up your metabolism. We know that if you don't understand why something works, you won't be motivated to try it. For instance, you will understand *why* you must become a devotee of breakfast.

We had a great way to prove our theories—and we took advantage of it. Each chapter contains a "twin trial." There are many things twins can do that no one else can.

For example, you can make your other half be a guinea pig for you. If you don't like what happens to your twin, then you don't follow in her footsteps. A few years ago, Tammy watched as a hairdresser got scissors-happy. She chopped Lyssie's long locks, which had hung halfway down her back, to hair that barely reached her earlobes. Lyssie's heart sank as she looked in the mirror with horror—the bobbed hair was far from flattering. On this particular day, Tammy happened to be the lucky one; she immediately noticed that this short hair was not a good look for us and decided that she would skip the chop.

When it came to writing this book, both of us fought to avoid being the guinea pig. When it comes to nutrition and exercising, we both practice what we preach because we like to do what makes us feel healthy—that makes us feel good. We realize that eating any other way won't allow us to feel our best. Our first twin experiment, which involved manipulating the carbohydrates we eat, caused quite a battle, as neither of us wanted to be the one to mess with the body's major fuel source.

However, despite the tension caused by the first trial, we continued to test each of these nine principles, one of us serving as a control, and one of us serving as a guinea pig. We are extremely regimented (almost to a fault, if you ask our mom), but this made us excellent study subjects, as we both eat the same amount of calories and foods. We have the same jobs and exercise together. Therefore, we could run trials in which the twin who was the guinea pig would not follow the recommendations of one of our basic premises. We saw the results—and they were dramatic!

You may wonder why we tested the nine principles, which people already seem to know about. But the truth is, they just don't get it. And until we saw the results of our trials, we weren't aware of how much each principle completely affects metabolism.

In addition, we conducted these trials because we didn't just want to tell you what to do. We wanted to prove to you why our tips will fire up your metabolism. People always make the mistake of thinking that they can lose weight only if they make drastic changes. We wanted to prove to you that making small changes, like any of the tips based on our nine simple principles, will fire up your metabolism and cause lasting weight loss more than anything else.

Whether you have tried every possible trick to lose body fat or have never tried in your life, whether you travel frequently or spend most of the day at your desk, this book will help you. We give you hundreds of specific suggestions and show you how to incorporate them. We help you time your meals and offer dozens of ideas for what to eat so that you're neither hungry nor craving metabolism-slowing foods. We also provide sample menus to help on the frontlines of your metabolic revolution.

Hundreds of tips is a lot. We include that many because we want you to choose which ones suit you best. You don't have to take advantage of every tip to see results.

If, however, you like to follow a step-by-step plan, we've got that for you, too.

So no matter who you are and what works best for your lifestyle, this book is designed to help you succeed.

Each chapter includes our clients' success stories. You will be inspired by how our clients gave their metabolism a jolt and not only saw mind boggling results but also changed their lives in other important ways. You, too, will experience this.

You will feel rejuvenated.

You will be more energetic and light on your feet.

Physical challenges such as staying alert in the afternoon, or walking up several flights of stairs, or running a couple of city blocks will be so easy that you won't give them a second thought.

Life will be easier. Everything from meeting your health and fitness goals to advancing in your career to having successful relationships with family, friends, and significant others will seem like less of a struggle.

Looking in the mirror will be enjoyable, and you will want to show off your new body.

People will compliment you.

You will have a newfound confidence.

You will have the knowledge and the motivation to have a completely fulfilled life.

Do You Have a Slow Metabolism?

TAKE THIS TEST AND FIND OUT

1. Do you have a hard time losing weight?   yes___ no___

2. Do you gain weight more easily than you
   lose it?   yes___ no___

3. Do you frequently skip breakfast?   yes___ no___

4. Do you often skip other meals? yes___ no✓___

5. Do you often wait longer than five hours between meals/snacks? yes___ no✓___

6. Do you often sit down to one or several large meals a day? yes✓___ no___

7. Do you often feel sleepy after a meal? yes✓___ no___

8. Do you usually finish everything on your plate? yes✓___ no___

9. Do you sleep fewer than seven hours a night? yes___ no✓___

10. Some days, do you feel much more tired than others, despite getting an adequate night's rest? yes✓___ no___

11. Do you often feel sluggish? yes___ no✓___

12. Do you often almost doze off at your desk after eating lunch? yes___ no✓___

13. Do you often have restless nights because of indigestion or feelings of fullness from eating too close to bedtime? yes___ no✓___

14. When you eat carbohydrates, do you usually choose pasta, white rice, white bread, and other refined carbohydrates? yes✓___ no___

15. Do you drink fewer than eight 8-ounce glasses of water a day? yes___ no✓___

16. Do you drink more than three alcoholic beverages a week? yes___ no✓___

17. Do you usually choose full-fat cheese, milk, yogurt, and other dairy products? yes___ no✓___

18. Do you frequently eat cookies, cakes, and candies? yes___ no✓___

19. Do you regularly use butter, lard, sour cream, or cream cheese? yes ✓ no___

20. Do you eat fried foods more than twice a week? yes___ no ✓

21. Do you exercise fewer than five times per week and/or fewer than thirty minutes per session? yes ✓ no___

22. Do you lift weights fewer than three times per week? yes___ no ✓

23. Do you often try popular diets? yes___ no ✓

24. Do you frequently lose weight and then gain it back? yes___ no ✓

25. Do you rarely get hunger pangs even if it has been many hours since you last ate? yes___ no ✓

26. Is your skin either very dry or very oily? yes___ no ✓

27. Are you apple-shaped (excess abdominal fat) rather than pear-shaped (excess hip, thigh, and buttocks fat)? yes___ no ✓

28. Are you impatient? yes___ no ✓

29. Do you have mood swings more than two times a month? yes___ no ✓

30. After eating sweets, do you frequently crave more? yes___ no ✓

31. Do your nails break or peel easily, or have grooves or yellow or white spots? yes ✓ no___

32. Are you very sensitive to heat or cold? yes ✓ no___

33. Does your body seem to change in an undesirable way with every passing year? yes ✓ no___

34. Do you sometimes feel as though you could eat all day long? yes ✓ no___

35. Do you eat more than usual when in social situations (with friends, at cocktail parties, etc.)? yes___ no _✓

36. Does your weight generally fluctuate by more than five pounds over the course of six months? yes___ no _✓

37. Do you eat fish less than once a week? yes _✓ no___

38. Have any of your family members, including grandparents and parents, had any of the following diseases/conditions?

High cholesterol	yes___	no _✓
High blood pressure	yes___	no _✓
Heart disease	yes___	no _✓
Stroke	yes _✓	no___
Diabetes	yes _✓	no___
Cancer	yes___	no _✓
Obesity	yes___	no _✓

39. Do you take any medication regularly, including birth control pills? yes _✓ no___

40. Do you sometimes forget to take your vitamins, or not take them at all? yes _✓ no___

41. Do you frequently drink juice, Gatorade, or other caloric beverages? yes___ no _✓

Now score yourself. Count your yes answers.

0–6: Excellent! Your metabolism has not slowed at this point. You are probably like us, who practice our Fire Up Your Metabolism tips regularly. However, as you will see in our twin trials, a lifetime of good work can easily go bad when our major principles are not applied, even for a short period of time. So use this book as a guide to help you to make sure that you are consistently revving your metabolism forever. You certainly do not need to follow the entire plan to fire up your metabolism. You can simply take advantage of as few as 10 percent of the tips that you aren't following now and really fire up your metabolism to its ultimate potential.

7–14: Although you have not drastically slowed your metabolism, it is not working as efficiently as it could be. You may be like our client Dawn, who considers herself health conscious. Dawn avoids fried foods and limits metabolism doozies like butter and rich meat. She tries to include fiber in her diet—she eats oatmeal and fruits and vegetables. Dawn rarely skips a meal, unless an unusual situation comes up at work and she simply doesn't have time. Like Dawn, you may go out to eat a couple of times a week and realize that it is harder to control exactly what you eat when you eat out; however, you still do your best. And like Dawn, you may have a job where you rarely get up from your desk, so you aim to get to the gym at least five to six times a week (although occasionally social situations get in the way of good intentions). And you may not get enough sleep.

Or perhaps you are more like Mark. Mark has the best intentions for his health, too. However, he is very social and occasionally has a couple of drinks with the guys and sometimes overeats at restaurants. Heart disease runs in his family, and he tries to protect his health by working out frequently and avoiding foods that have a lot of saturated fat, such as full-fat dairy products, baked goods, and fatty meats. He also makes sure never to skip a meal.

So like Mark and Dawn, you have the best intentions for your health, but you could be burning more calories and fat than you are. If you take advantage of 20 percent of the tips that you are not currently incorporating into your life, or if you follow the plan, you can fire up your metabolism to its ultimate potential.

15–26: Your metabolism is slowed and your body is not burning fat and calories efficiently. Perhaps you skip meals too frequently, or space them out too much, or overeat. Or maybe you eat at restaurants and your choices are wreaking havoc on your metabolism.

Perhaps you are inconsistent—some days you eat plenty of fruits and vegetables and whole grains, non- or low-fat dairy products, and lean meats; then other days you give in completely to your cravings and end up consuming fries and brownies. Or maybe you have omitted an entire food group such as grains from your diet. Or maybe you've grown so accustomed to snacking and grabbing a soda that you've completely forgotten about meals and water.

You might be like Tammy's husband, Scott, an athlete in high school and college. However, by the time he met Tammy, he had gained thirty pounds despite working out regularly. He thought he was in great shape, because he watched what he ate. Unfortunately, he didn't notice that he was choosing a lot of the wrong foods—refined carbohydrates such as white rice, bagels, muffins, white pasta, fatty cuts of steak, and ground turkey (which he actually thought was a health food).

Scott lost those thirty pounds quickly after meeting Tammy and learning about the principles of firing up his metabolism.

Although you may feel that you lead a healthy lifestyle, you have some metabolism-slowing habits. If you take advantage of thirty percent of the tips in this book, or if you follow the plan, you will dramatically speed up your metabolism every day, for the rest of your life.

27+: You are probably not at all surprised that your metabolism has been drastically slowed. You already know that you are burning far fewer calories and less fat than you should be. Chances are you have tried many diets in the past that may or may not have promoted weight loss, yet you probably have gained much of the weight back or find yourself as heavy as or heavier than ever.

Of course it's also possible that this is the first time you have taken steps to lose weight. Whichever scenario describes you, you are probably confused about what you should be eating. You may benefit the most by following the plan. However, if you are able to take advantage of 50 percent of the tips in this book that you don't currently follow, you will speed up your metabolism now and for the rest of your life.

ONE

Get Ready, Get Set, Get Fired Up

Now is the time to fire up your metabolism . . . and you will do it.

We are about to arm you with weapons that will reshape your body. Your metamorphosis will be effortless and simple. For now your only job is to believe in yourself. Know that you can do this. Know that you can follow the simple tips in our plan. The rest is in our hands as we help you fire up your metabolism.

Sound too easy? Well, ironically, the biggest obstacle for dieters is not their cravings but rather their lack of faith in themselves.

They don't believe that they will get through the tough times, and so they don't really try. People fall off their plan one day and grow discouraged.

As we said in the introduction, you don't have to be perfect in order to fire up your metabolism.

You are *not* going on a diet.

Instead, you are tweaking your habits to incorporate metabolism-revving tips. When you do, you *will see results.*

There are four things you must do to ensure your success. Don't cheat yourself by skipping the next four steps. This is the one time you're not allowed to cheat.

1. Avoid Overwhelming Your Metabolism: Learn What a Portion Looks Like

When we set different amounts of pasta or chicken in front of our clients and ask them which constitutes a serving, they commit portion distortion. In their heads, portion sizes appear bigger than they actually are—a 1-cup serving is regularly mistaken for being only ½ cup, and a ½-cup serving is thought to be only ¼ cup.

We live in a supersized society, where everything from beverages to snacks to bagels is overstuffed. In fact, restaurant portions are so enormous that we don't even know what a "normal" serving size looks like anymore. When we are served only the amount of food that our body needs, the restaurant appears stingy.

Thus, it is essential that you measure out ½ cup and 1 cup of cooked pasta or rice at least once a month, as "portion distortion" accrues over time. Place each portion on a plate so that you visualize exactly what it looks like. This does not mean that you can eat only ½ cup or 1 cup at a sitting, but you must know what ½ cup and 1 cup look like. (Remember, there are 8 ounces in 1 cup.)

Measuring takes only seconds. We promise.

Rice and pasta "bulk up" as they cook. Rice increases to three times its size, so ⅓ cup of raw rice equals 1 cup of cooked rice. Even though pasta comes in different shapes, as a general rule, 2 ounces raw equals ½ cup cooked.

When your body can't effectively burn up all of the food you have eaten, it becomes overwhelmed and stores the excess food as fat, usually on your stomach, hips, and thighs. You can "overwhelm" your metabolism by overeating certain foods.

2. The "Rule of Hand"

We live in a society where most people would describe their lives as hectic. As a result, the majority of us eat at least one meal per day away from home. Using measuring utensils to portion food is unrealistic.

What's more, restaurant plates are not the same size as those at home, which can exacerbate portion distortion.

Your hand plays a critical role when it comes to metabolism. Your hand will help you estimate portion sizes of specific foods.

a small woman's fist = 1 cup of cooked pasta or rice

a man's fist = 1½ cups cooked pasta or rice

food that fits in the cup of your hand = ½ cup

3 middle fingers = 2 ounces of lean meat

To use the Rule of Hand, simply place your fist or fingers next to the food you plan to eat and see how the food portion compares. If the food portion is bigger than the amount you had planned to eat at this meal, push the excess to the side of your plate. If you know you will be tempted to eat the extra food, put it on a bread plate and immediately ask your server to doggy-bag it or take it away.

3. The Food Diary

Tracking what you eat makes you aware of what you are actually eating. When you see the list of foods that you have consumed written down, you will either feel shocked or proud. (A sample food diary is on pages 42 and 43 in Chapter 2.)

You will also ensure your success by tracking your fitness progress in an exercise and strength-training journal. Just like with the food diary, you will see what you are and are not doing. (You will find the exercise journal on page 223 of Chapter 10 and the strength-training journal on page 239 of Chapter 11.)

These journals are the key to your metabolic revolution. Frequently, people who believe that they have made the appropriate changes to lose weight are unsuccessful. When they examine their journal, they are shocked to see that they didn't take as many steps toward their goal as they had thought. Your journals are your proof that you are taking the proper steps to guarantee your success. If you see that you aren't getting the necessary exercise or food, you will step it up.

4. One Last Thing to Guarantee Your Success

No one can take care of your body for you. Only *you control you.* Only you have the power over your body. Although we believe in you, and we know that you *will* succeed and *will* fire up your metabolism, now it is your turn. Remind yourself, *aloud,* several times each day that you will succeed. *Know* that *you* can do it. *Know* that you will succeed. Remember how disciplined and powerful you can be. Strategically place affirmations where you frequently look—your desk drawer at work, your bathroom mirror, your refrigerator, and your wallet. Be relentless about saying the affirmations several times a day. (If there is someone around and you are embarrassed to read the affirmations aloud, say them to yourself.)

It takes ten positive reinforced statements to counteract one negative statement. Write out ten affirmations that you will read aloud morning, noon, and night, to reiterate how strong you are and how successful you will be. Here are a few affirmations to get you started, but add your own, too.

- Today I am taking steps to make my metabolism into a well-oiled machine.

- Every day I will keep a food diary, an exercise journal, and a strength-training journal so that I can track my progress and be motivated by even the smallest achievement.

- I will reach my goal because I am allowing my body to burn more calories by not skipping breakfast today. I won't be hungry at 10 A.M. anymore, so I won't eat a piece of coffee cake in the midmorning.

- I'm going to be successful because I eat in a way that will rev up my metabolism.

- I am choosing a lifestyle that will lead to a body that burns calories extremely efficiently.

- I choose carbohydrates that are best for my metabolism.

- The proteins I choose are good choices, which keep me satiated and make me healthy. My immunity is high, my skin is healthy, my hair is shiny, and I feel lighter.

- I choose fats that make my blood run smoothly through my body and help my body to run efficiently. I am speeding up my metabolism.

- I am doing everything in my power to fire up my metabolism.

- I will reach my optimal weight by eating in a way that is healthy and will speed up my metabolism.

- I will wait no more than five hours between my meals/snacks.

- I will stick to a regular exercise and strength-training program.

- I will set short- and long-term achievable health goals for myself and do everything in my power to obtain them.

- I will shut off the TV a half hour before I go to bed so that I won't get distracted and stay up later than I should. This way I will go to bed earlier and sleep more so that the amount of sleep I get will positively affect my metabolism.

Before coming to see us, Carmine wholeheartedly set out to try one new diet after another. After a few days, however, she would put on a pair of pants or a shirt that still felt tight and look in the mirror and say, "What's the use? I'm never going to lose all this weight." Then she would feel helpless, give up, and go and eat a doughnut, or four. Carmine was never able to stay on a diet because her negative self overtook her goals.

Now when Carmine looks in the mirror, she sees positive affirmations that she will succeed. The notes say:

- Every day I apply the Rule of Hand and my body is burning calories more efficiently.

- Every day when I choose to eat oatmeal rather than Special K, I am taking control of my metabolism and I will be successful.

- I will reach my goal because I am allowing my body to burn more calories because I didn't skip breakfast today.

Carmine smothered herself in positive affirmations so that she realized that with every little step she took, she was gaining more and more control over her metabolism and her weight. Carmine ultimately lost sixty pounds and has kept it off for the past two years. Much of her success lies in her ability to believe in herself.

Small Steps Make Lasting Results

How Much Weight Can I Expect to Lose Each Week?

A safe and healthy weight loss is one to two pounds a week. Much more than that is not fat loss, but muscle and water weight loss. Your body is about 60 percent water, so you can lose a lot of water weight, but it is easily regained as soon as you eat or drink. As you will learn in the following chapters, muscle weight is not the weight you want to lose—losing muscle dramatically slows your metabolism since muscle burns calories.

You may know someone who has gone on a very strict diet and lost seven to ten pounds in the first week. This is not healthy and, in most cases, is not permanent. Initial weight loss is encouraging, but it is misleading—it actually slows your metabolism. As a basic rule, when it comes to weight loss, the quicker you lose it (more than three pounds per week), the quicker you gain it back.

TWO

Mixing Nutrients to Maximize Metabolism

Carbohydrates. Carbohydrates are the key to a speedy metabolism because they provide your body with the energy to be active. They are found in grains, such as pasta, rice, and bread; fruits and vegetables; dairy products (especially yogurt and milk); and beans. Beans and dairy products are also good sources of protein. (Note: Only yogurt and beans can be considered either carbs or protein.)

Carbs are critical for a speedy metabolism because all movements, even small ones, burn up calories. When you have a lot of energy, you are more likely to make many movements, and the more calories you'll burn. Remember, the more calories you burn, the faster your metabolism.

Protein. Eggs, meat, poultry, and fish contain protein. Soybeans and products such as tofu, soy milk, and other foods made from soybeans are also rich in protein. Beans and dairy products are good sources of protein, too. Nuts and seeds provide substantial amounts of protein, but they contain large amounts of fat and therefore fall in the "fat" category. Protein is key to a speedy metabolism because it helps you to build lean muscle, which helps burn calories quickly. The more muscle you have, the faster your metabolism.

Fats. Oils, cream, butter, olives, nuts, seeds, mayonnaise, salad dressings, and avocados are considered fats. Although all animal products such as meat, fish, poultry, and all dairy products (without the fat removed) contain fat, meat, milk, cheese, and yogurt fall in the protein category because they provide large amounts of protein. Likewise, although sweets such as cookies and cakes often have a lot of added fat, we include these foods on the carbohydrate lists. Fats are important to metabolism because they slow the digestion of the carbohydrates and allow for more sustained energy, which keeps your body active longer so you burn more calories.

Maximize Your Metabolic Fire: Choose the Best Carbohydrates, Protein, and Fats, and Mix Them Together Appropriately

When it comes to your metabolism, carbohydrates, protein, and fats play unique roles. You need to eat foods from all of the groups. Carbohydrates cannot replace the role of protein or fat; fat and protein cannot replace each other or carbohydrates.

And even if you are eating the right amounts of these nutrients, there is something you may not know: *Choosing just any protein, or randomly picking any fat or carbohydrate, will not fire up your metabolism.* You must choose the best foods in these categories to prevent cravings and overeating, and most important, to enhance your body's ability to utilize energy and burn calories, thus speeding up your metabolism.

For instance, by choosing to eat 1 cup of brown rice with 3 ounces (size of a deck of cards) of grilled turkey breast instead of 1 cup of white rice and 3 ounces of *ground* turkey, you will positively affect your metabolic rate.

As you read this book, you will probably be surprised to learn which nutrients are actually responsible for firing up your metabolic engine and which are critical for burning more calories for a longer time. You don't have to worry about counting or calculating the proportions. Just follow our simple tips—we have done the work for you.

All of your meals and snacks will consist of the best carbohydrates with adequate portions of the most beneficial proteins and/or fats. This should be nothing new for you—in fact, you probably eat carbohydrates with proteins or fats most of the time. For example, when you eat a turkey sandwich, you are eating carbohydrates (bread) with modest amounts of protein (turkey). And when you eat cereal with milk, the cereal provides you with ample carbohydrates while the milk offers a good source of protein. The only difference is that now we will help to ensure that you are choosing the *best* carbohydrates, proteins, and fats in the appropriate proportions.

Eating the Unthinkable?

Carbohydrates are in the hot seat. As a consumer, you have heard it all. First, you hear you want a diet high in carbs, then you hear that you want a diet low in carbs, and then, just as you feel utterly confused, you hear that if you want to lose weight you should eat a diet with no carbs. What is the scoop on carbohydrates—those foods you love to love yet that many popular diet books love to hate? Well, forget what you've heard. Here's the real deal.

You *can* eat carbs and lose weight.

In fact, you *should* eat carbs because they provide your body with energy to burn calories. You can even eat a cookie, pasta, or a roll with dinner without guilt. Although these are not the best carbohydrates to choose, you don't have to swear off them.

Carbs fuel your muscles, central nervous system, and red blood cells. Without them you won't have energy. Without energy, you will become too lethargic to engage in activity. You will even conserve energy by cutting back on the smallest of movements (for instance, you won't get up out of your office chair as frequently, or when you are standing, you'll lean on something rather than support your own weight), and you'll hardly burn a calorie.

You will be exhausted and conserve energy every chance you get. The resulting inactivity will lead to weight gain. So even small amounts of carbohydrates must be part of *every* meal in order to give you a continuous energy boost throughout the day.

Some carbs are much better than others. We've broken them down into three groups: "always" carbs should constitute over half of your daily calorie intake and should be chosen nine out of ten times you have carbs; "sometimes" carbs should be limited, not chosen more than two times out of ten; and "rarely" carbs should be saved for special occasions and eaten no more than one out of every ten times you eat a carb. It's imperative to learn which are which.

"Always" Carbs are made from whole grains and include unrefined plant foods—vegetables, fruits, and legumes. They take a long time to digest, which makes them metabolism-friendly.

They provide ample carbohydrate with little or no fat. In theory, these plant foods (carbohydrates) are as good as it gets—wholesome food grown straight from the soil, the child of our very own Mother Nature. Changed minimally, if at all, by the time they reach our plates, they are so nutritious that the American Heart Association and the American Diabetes Association recommend eating more whole grains, fruits, vegetables, and beans, all of which are carbohydrates. And the National Cancer Institute recommends that we get at least five servings of fruits and vegetables a day. (Some new research shows that we should get twice this—ten servings a day.)

Carbs that are rich in fiber—such as brown rice, oatmeal, whole wheat bread, Raisin Bran, and fruits, vegetables, and beans—can take as long as two to four hours to digest because the fiber slows digestion. As a result, you feel full longer, and your body receives a longer-lasting supply of energy. The longer your body is energized, the more active you will be, and the more calories you will burn.

BUYER BEWARE: Just because the bread is darker in color doesn't mean it's whole wheat; it may just mean that caramel color has been added. Be sure to read the ingredients label.

"Sometimes" and "Rarely" Carbs include white rice, white bread, cookies, candies, and cake. These foods have been so processed that their nutrients and fiber are gone by the time they get to you.

Usually the fiber is replaced with metabolically detrimental ingredients, like sugar and additives. You digest these processed "sometimes" and "rarely" carbs so quickly that you get a sugar "high," only to be followed by a "crash." This energy low causes the brain to signal that it needs more fuel (food) so that it can get some energy. You turn to the food that will provide you with energy the fastest—sugar and more refined "sometimes" and "rarely" carbohydrates. The bad news, of course, is that your brain is craving food even though you have just eaten. That's overeating.

"Always" carbs, conversely, keep energy levels stable, which in turn prevents sugar highs and crashes and, most important, the subsequent overeating and inevitable weight gain.

We know it's not always easy to find "always" carbs. Processed food is everywhere. However, by simply learning which carbohydrates you should "always" choose, and which you should "sometimes" and "rarely" choose, it will be easy for you to recognize your best metabolism-revving choices. You will be able to locate an "always" carbohydrate almost anywhere you go, and the good news is that all vegetables and all fruits (unless they are canned in syrup) are "always" carbohydrates.

So grains, not fruits and vegetables, can fall under the less desirable categories. Keep your eye on these. Be sure to choose the "always" grains nine times out of ten times that you eat a grain serving.

"Always" Carbohydrates

If you don't see your favorite grain on the "always" list, simply check the label for its ingredients—the first ingredient must be "whole-grain" flour. For bread to be 100 percent whole wheat, "whole wheat flour" should be the only flour listed.

"Wheat," "enriched," or "unbleached" flours are refined flours and are *not* part of the "always" list. Don't be fooled. "Wheat" bread is refined and processed. Seven-grain, nine-grain, and twelve-grain breads usually are not "always" carbohydrates either; they are usually made from refined "sometimes" carbohydrates and sprinkled with a few whole grains, but in insignificant amounts. See pages 63 to 66 to determine how many servings of carbohydrates you personally need each day to fire up your metabolism. Specified portions of grains are equivalent to one serving from the grain/carbohydrate group.

You do not need to eat only one portion of the listed carbohydrate at one sitting. However, if you are following the plan and not just the tips, you do need to make sure that you know how many portions you eat over the course of the day so that you do not overeat your daily requirement. See pages 65 and 66 in order to determine how many servings of carbohydrate you need to fire up your metabolism.

All fruits and vegetables come straight from the ground, are not processed, and are packed with fiber, vitamins, minerals, and disease-fighting phytochemicals. Choose fresh and frozen over canned vegetables; frozen is just as nutritious as fresh, but canned vegetables have added sodium and have lost some nutrients in the water they are canned in.

To determine if a grain is an "always," "sometimes," or "rarely" carbohydrate, ask yourself how far removed it is from the ground. In other words, how similar is the carbohydrate to the way it grew from the soil? Has it been picked apart? Have fiber and nutrients been removed? Have sugar and other fillers been added?

The product has not been plucked apart, its nutrients are intact, and it is similar to the way it grew in the ground if it lists "whole wheat" or "whole grain" first on the ingredient label or if the front label says "100% whole wheat" or "100% whole grain." Grains that have been processed and are farther removed from the ground say "wheat," "white," "unbleached flour," or "enriched flour" on the ingredients label—they are "sometimes" and "rarely" carbohydrates. Also, you can use our list on pages 23 to 31 to see which foods qualify.

"ALWAYS" CARBOHYDRATES

Specified portions are equal to one serving.

Beans*, ¹/₂ cup (all beans and bean soups, with the exception of baked beans with bacon or lard and refried beans)

Breads

> **English muffin, oat bran,** ¹/₂ muffin
>
> **English muffin, whole wheat,** ¹/₂ muffin
>
> **Matzo,** Manischewitz 100% whole wheat, 1 piece
>
> **Pita,** whole wheat, ¹/₂ of large pita
>
> **Pumpernickel** (label must say "whole" pumpernickel), 1 slice
>
> **Tortilla,** whole wheat, 6" diameter, 1
>
> **Whole grain rye,** 1 slice
>
> **Whole wheat,** 1 slice
>
> **Whole wheat, reduced calorie,** 2 slices
>
> **Bun,** whole wheat, ¹/₂ bun

Breakfast Grains: Pancakes and Waffles

> **Pancakes, whole wheat,** 4" diameter, 1
>
> **Pancakes, whole wheat (Arrowhead Mills),** 4" diameter, 1
>
> **Pancakes, whole wheat (Aunt Jemima**—although not entirely whole wheat, it is more whole wheat than white flour), 4" diameter, 1
>
> **Waffles (Eggo Nutri-Grain Multigrain),** 1 waffle
>
> **Waffles (Van's 7 Grain Whole Wheat**—one of the few times when seven-grain is 100 percent whole grain!), 1 waffle

Cereals: Specified portions of cereals are equal to one serving from the grain group. "Always" cereals are the whole grains; they are unprocessed and unrefined, and they have more than three grams of fiber and fewer than nine grams of sugar per serving.

> **All-Bran, extra fiber,** 1 cup
>
> **All-Bran, original,** ³/₄ cup
>
> **Bran Flakes (Post),** ³/₄ cup
>
> **Cheerios,** plain, 1 cup
>
> **Chex, Multi-Bran,** ¹/₂ cup
>
> **Chex, Wheat,** ²/₃ cup
>
> **Fiber One,** 1 cup
>
> **Frosted Mini-Wheats (Kellogg's),** 3 biscuits

Frosted Mini-Wheats Bite Size Cereal (Kellogg's), 12 biscuits

Granola, low-fat, no sugar added, 1/4 cup

Grape-Nuts Flakes, 3/4 cup

Grape-Nuts, 1/4 cup

Honey Frosted Mini-Wheats, 12 biscuits

Kashi Go Lean, 3/4 cup

Kashi Good Friends, 1 cup

Kashi, Puffed, seven-whole-grain and sesame, 1 1/3 cups

Life, 3/4 cup

Muesli, 1/3 cup

Nutri-Grain, corn, 2/3 cup

Nutri-Grain, wheat, 2/3 cup

Nutri-Grain Golden Wheat (Kellogg's), 3/4 cup

Oat bran hot cereal, 1/2 cup, cooked

Oatmeal, instant or slow-cooked, regular (Quaker), 1/2 cup, cooked

Raisin Bran (Kellogg's and Post), 1/2 cup

Raisin Bran (Total), 2/3 cup

Ralston 100% Wheat hot cereal, 1/2 cup, cooked

Roman Meal, 1/2 cup, cooked

Shredded Wheat (Post), 2/3 cup or 1 1/2 large biscuits

Shredded Wheat N' Bran (Post), 2/3 cup

Total, 3/4 cup

Wheatena, 1/2 cup, cooked

Wheaties, 1 cup

Wheaties, Energy Crunch, 1/2 cup

Crackers

Ak-Mak, 5 slices

Health Valley Whole Wheat (low fat), 10 crackers

Ry Krisp, 3 crackers

Wasa Organic Rye Original Crispbread, 4 slices

Wasa Original Whole Wheat Crispbread, 2 slices

Fruits: The number of fruit servings you need is equal to the number of fat servings you need. See pages 73 to 74, Chapter 3, to determine your personal requirement.

Apple, 1 small

Applesauce, unsweetened, 1/2 cup

Apricots, 4

Banana, 1 small or $\frac{1}{2}$ large

Blackberries, $\frac{1}{2}$ cup

Blueberries, $\frac{1}{2}$ cup

Cantaloupe, $\frac{1}{2}$ whole or 1 cup cubed

Cherries, $\frac{3}{4}$ cup

Grapefruit, $\frac{1}{2}$ large or 1 small

Grapes, 15 grapes or $\frac{3}{4}$ cup

Honeydew, 1 wedge ($\frac{1}{8}$ of melon) or 1 cup cubed

Kiwi, $1\frac{1}{2}$

Mango, $\frac{1}{2}$ large

Nectarine, 1 large

Orange, 1 large

Peach, 1 large

Pear, 1 small

Pineapple, $\frac{1}{2}$ cup chunks

Raisins, $\frac{1}{4}$ cup

Strawberries, $\frac{1}{2}$ cup sliced or 1 cup whole

Watermelon, 1 cup cubed

Grains

Barley, $\frac{1}{2}$ cup cooked

Buckwheat groats (kasha), $\frac{1}{2}$ cup cooked

Bulgur, whole grain, $\frac{1}{2}$ cup cooked

Quinoa, $\frac{1}{2}$ cup cooked

Rice, brown, $\frac{1}{2}$ cup cooked

Pasta, whole wheat, $\frac{1}{2}$ cup cooked

Popcorn and Pretzels

Popcorn, air-popped, 3 cups

Popcorn (Bearitos, No Salt, No Oil), 4 cups popped

Popcorn (Healthy Choice), 6 cups popped

Popcorn (Pop Secret, Light), 5 cups popped

Pretzels, whole wheat, 1 large

Vegetables: You should eat *at least* $4\frac{1}{2}$ vegetable servings a day. Eating more than $4\frac{1}{2}$ servings of any vegetable is encouraged, with the exception of peas, potatoes, and corn, which are too high in starch to be eaten in unlimited amounts. You will find the serving sizes for the starchy vegetables on the list below.

Corn, 1 medium ear or ¹/₂ cup

Peas (starchy vegetable, so it counts as a grain), ¹/₂ cup

Potato, white or sweet, flesh and skin, baked, 3 ounces (about 4" long)

Tomatoes, cherry or grape, ¹/₂ cup

Vegetables, cooked, ¹/₂ cup

Vegetables, raw, chopped, ¹/₂ cup

Vegetables, raw, leafy, 1 cup

Yogurt

Yogurt*, low-fat, fruit added with low-calorie sweetener, ¹/₂ cup

Yogurt*, nonfat, plain, 1 cup

Yogurt*, nonfat, sugar-free, 1 cup

---

*Can be counted as a carbohydrate serving or a protein serving.

"Sometimes" Carbohydrates

These are made with refined flour. The ingredient list on the label says "enriched wheat flour," "bromated flour," or "rice flour." Choose a "sometimes" carbohydrate (grain) only when its "always" counterpart is not available. For instance, if you are at a restaurant and would like to eat pasta, the "always" carbohydrate would be whole wheat pasta. Most restaurants don't serve whole wheat pasta, so you may have to choose the "sometimes" carbohydrate regular pasta. *Eat these "sometimes" grains a maximum of two times out of ten, or one time out of ten if you are also having one "rarely" grain serving.*

Love that seven- or nine-grain bread but disappointed because yours turns out not to be made from the whole grain? Try Bakers brand bread, sold at health food stores and many supermarkets. Its seven-grain and nine-grain breads actually are made with the whole grain.

"SOMETIMES" CARBOHYDRATES

Specified portions are equivalent to one serving.

Bagels (even whole wheat bagels—whole wheat is not the first ingredient in whole wheat bagels, they just get a sprinkle of unrefined flour), 3" diameter, ½

Breads

    Bun, hamburger, ½ bun

    Crushed or cracked wheat, 1 slice

    English muffin, raisin or plain, ½ muffin

    French, 1 slice

    Honey wheat, 1 slice

    Italian, 1 slice

    Multigrain, 1 slice

    Oatmeal, 1 slice

    Olive, 1 slice

    Pumpernickel (label must say "whole" pumpernickel to make it an "always" carb), 1 slice

    Rye (if "whole" rye is the first ingredient on the label, then it is an "always" carb), 1 slice

    Seven-grain or nine-grain (usually just sprinkled with the unrefined flour, most is processed), 1 slice

    Sunflower, 1 slice

    Tortilla, flour, 6" diameter, 1

    White, 1 slice

Cereal bar (Health Valley Bakes or Healthy Breakfast Bakes), 1 bar

Cereals: Specified portions of cereals are equal to one serving from the grain group. "Sometimes" cereals (such as flavored Cheerios and Quaker instant flavored oatmeal) are either whole grains with too much added sugar to be on the "always" list, or they are not the whole grain; however, they are low in fat and have between ten and fifteen grams of sugar per serving.

    Alpha-Bits, ¾ cup

    Basic 4, ½ cup

    Cheerios, Apple Cinnamon (too high in sugar to be on the "always" list), ¾ cup

Cheerios, Frosted (too high in sugar to be on the "always" list), $^3/_4$ cup

Cheerios, Honey Nut (too high in sugar to be on the "always" list), $^3/_4$ cup

Chex, Corn, 1 cup

Chex, Rice, 1 cup

Cinnamon Toast Crunch, $^1/_2$ cup

Corn Flakes (Kellogg's), 1 cup

Cracklin' Oat Bran, $^1/_3$ cup

Cream of Rice, 1 instant packet or $^1/_2$ cup cooked

Cream of Wheat, 1 instant packet or $^1/_2$ cup cooked

Crispix, 1 cup

Frosted Flakes (Kellogg's), $^2/_3$ cup

Golden Grahams, $^1/_2$ cup

Granola (Kellogg's low-fat no raisins) (too high in sugar to be on the "always" list), $^1/_3$ cup

Granola (Kellogg's low-fat with raisins) (too high in sugar to be on the "always" list), $^1/_3$ cup

Grits, 1 packet instant or $^1/_2$ cup cooked

Harmony, Vanilla Almond Oat, $^2/_3$ cup

Honey Bunches of Oats, Honey Roasted, $^2/_3$ cup

Honeycomb, 1 cup

Just Right Fruit and Nut, $^1/_2$ cup

Kashi, Honey Puffed, 1 cup

Kashi Medley, $^1/_2$ cup

Kix, 1 cup

Life, Cinnamon, $^3/_4$ cup

Oatmeal, instant, flavored (Quaker) (too high in sugar to be on the "always" list), $^3/_4$ packet

Post Selects, Banana Nut Crunch, $^1/_2$ cup

Post Selects, Great Grains Crunchy Pecans, $^1/_4$ cup

Post Selects, Great Grains, Raisins, Dates, Pecans, $^1/_4$ cup

Product 19, 1 cup

Puffed Wheat (Quaker), $2^1/_4$ cups

Raisin Bran Crunch, $^1/_2$ cup

Rice Krispies (Kellogg's), 1 cup

Shredded Wheat, Frosted, $^2/_3$ cup

Smart Start, ¹/₂ cup

Special K, 1 cup

Special K with Strawberries, ³/₄ cup

Total, Brown Sugar and Oats, ³/₄ cup

Total Corn Flakes, 1¹/₃ cups

Chips, baked, ³/₄ ounce

Chips, soy, 15 chips

Crackers

Saltines, 8 crackers

Wheat Thins, 11 crackers

Croutons, ¹/₂ cup

Grains

Couscous, ¹/₂ cup

White rice, ¹/₂ cup cooked

Granola bar (Health Valley), 1 bar

Granola bar, low-fat chewy (Quaker), 1 bar

Pancakes, white flour, 4" diameter, 1

Pasta, ¹/₂ cup cooked

Pretzels, 1 ounce

Rice cakes, 2 large

Snack bar (Balance Outdoor Bar, Power Bar Harvest, or Performance), ¹/₂ bar

"Rarely" Carbohydrates

Just like "sometimes" carbs (grains), "rarely" carbs (grains) contain little fiber. However, "rarely" grains such as sugary candies and pastries aren't just low in fiber, they are also high in added sugar and/or fat, and therefore they have extra calories.

The "rarely" carbohydrates greatly hinder efforts to fire up your metabolism because they give your body a sugar high followed by an energy crash, which makes you less active and unable to burn many calories. When your body burns fewer calories, it is a sign that your metabolic rate has slowed. To make matters worse, the lows that these "rarely" carbs create leave you craving more food.

Although "rarely" carbs are not your metabolism's best friend, we don't recommend completely denying yourself these treats. Moderation is key to banishing that terrible feeling of deprivation that will lead to your giving in to temptation, which is exactly what we've witnessed with those who deny themselves the "rarely" carbohydrates: People inevitably wind up bingeing on these "treats." So limit your "rarely" grains by choosing them only once out of every ten times that you have a grain.

"RARELY" CARBOHYDRATES

Each specified portion is equal to one serving.

Biscuit, 1 small

Beverages
    Beer, 8 ounces
    Beer, light, 12 ounces
    Gatorade, 12 ounces
    Soda, regular, 8 ounces

Cake, $1/18$ of 8" x $3^{1}/2$" x $3^{1}/4$" cake ($1/2$ of slice)

Candy bar, $1/3$ of bar

Cereals: These are refined and processed and loaded with fat and/or sugar (14 or more grams of sugar per serving). These carbohydrates in the specified portions should be limited to one out of every ten times. Any sugar cereal marketed to kids, such as:
    Cap'n Crunch, all varieties, $3/4$ cup
    Cocoa Pebbles, $3/4$ cup
    Cocoa Puffs, 1 cup
    Cocoa Rice Krispies, $3/4$ cup
    Corn Pops, 1 cup
    Count Chocula, 1 cup
    Froot Loops, $3/4$ cup
    Fruity Pebbles, $3/4$ cup

Kellogg's Smacks, $^3/_4$ cup

Lucky Charms, 1 cup

Post Golden Crisp, $^3/_4$ cup

Post Selects, Blueberry Morning, $^1/_2$ cup

Trix, 1 cup

Chocolate candy, $^3/_4$ ounce

Croissant, $4^1/_2$" x 4" x $1^3/_4$", $^1/_2$ croissant

Doughnut, $3^1/_4$" diameter, $^1/_2$ doughnut

French fries, $^1/_2$ small order

Ice cream, $^1/_3$ cup

Jell-O (sugar added), $^1/_2$ cup

Muffin, $2^1/_2$" diameter, $1^1/_2$" high, 1 muffin

Pie, 9" diameter, $^1/_{24}$ of pie

Popcorn, Crunch'n Munch, $^1/_2$ cup

Pop-Tart, low-fat (Kellogg's), $^1/_2$ tart

Potato chips, $^3/_4$ ounce (about 11 chips)

Potato chips, fat free, made with Olestra, 1 ounce

Pudding, $^1/_3$ cup

Snack bar (Balance Gold), $^1/_2$ bar

Sugary candy, jelly beans, gummy candies, hard candies, 1 ounce

Toaster pastry, $^1/_2$ pastry

Yogurt, frozen, $^1/_2$ cup (fat-free is best)

Protein: Why You Should Combine It With Carbs to Get a Metabolic Boost

Protein has many important functions, but it does not give your body energy. Instead it slows the digestion of the carbohydrates and makes the energy and the metabolic boost from the carbohydrates last longer, which is why it is essential to mix carbohydrates with protein. So eating small amounts of protein with energy-boosting carbohydrates prevents hunger and extends the energy boost of the carbs.

However, eating a large portion of protein at one sitting will make you feel sluggish as blood rushes to your stomach and stays there, working to digest all of that protein. Your brain and muscles are left short on blood supply and energy. (Think about how you feel after a big steak dinner.)

To find out how many protein servings *you* need each day, see pages 65 and 66. The number of daily protein servings that you need to fire up your metabolism is equal to the number of grain servings you need. Also, see pages 73 to 74 to find out how many fruit servings you need. Every time you eat a carbohydrate, mix it with a protein. (There are a few exceptions that you will learn in this book. For instance, eating fruit by itself for an after-dinner snack is fine.)

Dairy products also contain some carbohydrates. However, when it comes to metabolism, the only dairy product we refer to as a carbohydrate is yogurt. Actually, both yogurt and legumes (beans) have a bonus—they can provide the benefits of both carbohydrates and proteins as they contain substantial amounts of both of these fuels. However, we discuss milk products other than yogurt in the protein chapter, as they provide substantial amounts of protein.

"THUMBS-UP" POWERFUL PROTEINS

Portion sizes are based on the average-size hand. If your hand is larger than average, then have $3/4$ of the recommended portion.

Do not have more than half of your daily servings at one sitting, or you will be left with too little food at your other meals. Your energy—and metabolism—will lag.

We have also included serving sizes for those of you who prefer to measure your foods.

FOOD	PORTION SIZE	RULE OF HAND
BEANS*		
All beans, with the exception of baked beans with bacon or lard and refried beans	$1/2$ cup	Fits into the cup of your hand
Edamame beans, with shells	$2/3$ cup	Covers both palms
EGGS		
Egg Beaters	$1/2$ cup	Fits into the cup of your hand
Egg whites	4	Fits into the cup of your hand
Hard-boiled	1	Fits into the cup of your hand
CHEESE		
Cottage, nonfat, low-fat, and 1%	$1/2$ cup	Fits into the cup of your hand
Feta	$3/4$ ounce	1 pointer finger
Goat (soft only)	$3/4$ ounce	1 pointer finger
Low-fat, all varieties (prepackaged slice)	$3/4$ ounce	1 pointer finger
Mozzarella, nonfat	1 ounce	$1 1/2$ pointer fingers
Mozzarella, part skim	$3/4$ ounce	1 pointer finger
Nonfat, all varieties	1 ounce	$1 1/2$ pointer fingers
Ricotta, low-fat	$1/3$ cup	Fills $1/2$ the cup of your hand
Ricotta, nonfat	$1/2$ cup	Fits into the cup of your hand
Soy cheese, nonfat	1 ounce	$1 1/2$ pointer fingers
Soy cheese, regular	$3/4$ ounce	1 pointer finger
Swiss, nonfat	1 ounce	$1 1/2$ pointer fingers

*Can be counted as either a carbohydrate serving or a protein serving.

CREAM

Sour cream, nonfat	1/4 cup	Fills 1/2 the cup of your hand

FISH/SEAFOOD
(all preparations except fried)

Bass	2 ounces	3 middle fingers
Clams, steamed, with shells	10	2 large handfuls
Cod	2 ounces	3 middle fingers
Crabmeat	2 ounces	3 middle fingers
Flounder	2 ounces	3 middle fingers
Grouper	2 ounces	3 middle fingers
Halibut	2 ounces	3 middle fingers
Lobster meat	1/2 cup	Fits into the cup of your hand
Oysters, without shells	1/3 cup	Covers the palm of your hand
Pollack	2 ounces	3 middle fingers
Salmon	2 ounces	3 middle fingers
Sardines	2 ounces	3 middle fingers
Scallops	2 ounces	3 middle fingers
Shrimp	5 shrimp (2 ounces)	Fits into the cup of your hand
Snapper	2 ounces	3 middle fingers
Squid	2 ounces	3 middle fingers
Swordfish	2 ounces	3 middle fingers
Tuna, canned, packed in water	2 ounces	3 middle fingers

MEATS

Bacon, Canadian only, patties	2 thin, round patties	3/4 of your palm
Bacon, Canadian only, strips	2 long slices	2 pointer fingers
Bacon, Canadian, extra-lean, patties	3 thin round patties	3/4 of your palm
Bacon, Canadian, extra-lean, strips	3 long slices	3 pointer fingers
Bacon, turkey	2 long slices	2 pointer fingers
Bacon, turkey, extra-lean	3 long slices	3 pointer fingers
Beef, bottom round, all fat removed	2 ounces	3 middle fingers

Beef, chuck, roasted, lean only	2 ounces	3 middle fingers
Beef, eye of round, all fat removed	2 ounces	3 middle fingers
Beef, ground, extra lean only	2 ounces	3 middle fingers
Beef, round tip, all fat trimmed	2 ounces	3 middle fingers
Beef, top loin, all fat removed	2 ounces	3 middle fingers
Beef, top sirloin, all fat removed	2 ounces	3 middle fingers
Ham, baked, lean only	2 ounces	3 middle fingers
Lamb chop, loin, lean only	2 ounces	3 middle fingers
Steak, broiled, extra-lean	$3/4$ ounces	1 pointer finger

MILK

Milk, nonfat	$3/4$ cup	$3/4$ of your fist
Milk, 1%	$3/4$ cup	$3/4$ of your fist
Soy milk, full-fat	$3/4$ cup	$3/4$ of your fist
Soy milk, low-fat	$3/4$ cup	$3/4$ of your fist

POULTRY

Chicken breast, not fried	2 ounces	3 middle fingers
Turkey breast, ground	2 ounces	3 middle fingers
Turkey breast, not fried	2 ounces	3 middle fingers

TOFU

Breakfast links (like Morningstar Farms)	2 links	2 pointer fingers
Breakfast patty (like Morningstar Farms)	1 patty	$3/4$ of your palm
Soy crumbles	$1/2$ cup	Fits into the cup of your hand
Tofu, baked or grilled	2 ounces	3 middle fingers
Veggie frank (like Natural Touch)	$3/4$ link	3 middle fingers
Veggie burger (like Boca Burger)	1 original-size burger; $3/4$ of bigger varieties	Size of your palm

YOGURT*

Low-fat, fruit added with low-calorie or regular sweetener	$1/2$ cup	Fits into the cup of your hand
Nonfat, fruit on the bottom	$3/4$ cup	Fills a little more than the cup of your hand
Nonfat, plain	1 cup	Size of your fist
Nonfat, sugar-free	1 cup	Size of your fist

Fat can bog down protein just like it does with carbs. Large amounts of artery-clogging fats make you lethargic. The less energy you have, the fewer movements you perform, and the fewer calories you burn. Therefore, these high-fat proteins get the thumbs-down. They are listed below in their *specified portions* and can be eaten seven times a week. You can have all seven servings in a splurge day, or you can have one serving every day.

"THUMBS-DOWN" PERILOUS PROTEINS

Choose only seven of the items below per week.

FOOD	PORTION SIZE	RULE OF HAND
BEANS		
Baked, with added bacon or lard	¼ cup	Fills ½ the cup of your hand
Refried	¼ cup	Fills ½ the cup of your hand
CHEESE made with whole milk		
Brie	¾ ounce	1 pointer finger
Cottage, whole and 2% fat	¼ cup	Fills ½ the cup of your hand
Goat cheese (hard and semihard)	½ ounce	1 pinkie
Gouda	½ ounce	1 pinkie
Mozzarella	¾ ounce	1 pointer finger
Parmesan, grated	½ ounce	1 pinkie
Swiss	¾ ounce	1 pointer finger
Swiss, part skim	¾ ounce	1 pointer finger
FISH/SEAFOOD		
Fried fish	¾ ounce	1 pointer finger
Squid, fried	¾ ounce	1 pointer finger
Tuna, canned, packed in oil	1 ounce	1½ pointer fingers
MEATS fatty cuts (red meat and pork), any fried meat, or meat with skin		
Bacon	1 piece	1 pointer finger
Beef, round, roasted, lean only	¾ ounce	1 pointer finger

Organ meats	$^3/_4$ ounce	1 pointer finger
Pork chop, lean, braised	$^3/_4$ ounce	1 pointer finger
Pork chop, lean and fat, braised	$^1/_2$ ounce	1 pinkie
Pork cutlet	$^1/_2$ ounce	1 pinkie
Prime rib, lean only	$^1/_2$ ounce	1 pinkie
Sausage	$^3/_4$ ounce	1 pointer finger
Steak, broiled, lean only	$^1/_2$ ounce	1 pinkie

MILK

Goat milk	$^1/_3$ cup	Fills $^3/_4$ the cup of your hand
Milk, 2%	$^1/_2$ cup	Fits into the cup of your hand
Milk, whole	$^1/_3$ cup	Fills $^3/_4$ the cup of your hand

POULTRY

Chicken drumstick	$^3/_4$ ounce	1 pointer finger
Chicken, fried, any part of bird	$^3/_4$ ounce	1 pointer finger
Chicken thigh	$^3/_4$ ounce	1 pointer finger
Chicken wing	$^3/_4$ ounce	1 pointer finger
Duck	$^3/_4$ ounce	1 pointer finger
Goose	$^3/_4$ ounce	1 pointer finger
Turkey, fried, any part of bird	$^1/_2$ ounce	1 pinkie
Turkey, ground, all parts	$^1/_2$ ounce	1 pinkie
Turkey gizzard	$^1/_2$ ounce	1 pinkie

YOGURT

Yogurt, plain, whole milk	$^1/_3$ cup	Fills $^3/_4$ the cup of your hand

Fat: Not the Metabolism Enemy You Think It Is— When You Mix It with Other Nutrients

You do need *some* fat.

When it comes to your metabolism, fat's function is crucial. It digests even more slowly than protein, and when you include it in your meals, you don't feel ravenous just a couple hours after eating. Therefore, fat helps to prevent overeating and bingeing. More important, when it comes to your metabolism, fat, like protein, has the ability to extend the energy-boosting and metabolism-revving effects of the

In the Fire Up Your Metabolism plan, your daily grain servings will equal your daily protein servings; likewise, your daily fat servings will equal your daily fruit servings. A key factor in jump-starting your metabolism is always to eat a grain carbohydrate serving with some fat or some protein.

carbohydrates by slowing the digestion of the carbohydrates and helping to provide more sustained energy (the more energy you have, the more activity you will perform and the more calories you will burn). Thus, you should mix fat with a carbohydrate, as fat plays a critical role in keeping the metabolism working in high gear.

Like protein, eating too much fat at one sitting backfires. Think of how drowsy you feel after an ice cream sundae or a gigantic portion of french fries.

At this point, you won't be surprised to learn that some fats are better than others. Animal fats, such as butter and poultry fat, for example, are fat "foes." As you will learn in this book, these fats in particular contribute to a slow metabolism. Limit these fat "foes" to a maximum of one a day—and try to replace them with "friendly" fats like nuts, olive oil, and avocados, which also are healthy for your heart.

Fats: What Equals One Fat Serving?

"FRIENDLY" FATS

FOOD	SERVING SIZE
FRUITS	
Avocado, mashed	¼ cup
NUTS AND SEEDS	
Almond butter	1 flat tablespoon
Almonds	14

Brazil nuts, unblanched	4
Cashew butter	1 flat tablespoon
Cashews, dry or oil roasted	11
Chestnuts, European, roasted	$\frac{1}{4}$ cup
Filberts/hazelnuts	11
Flaxseeds, ground	$2\frac{1}{2}$ tablespoons
Macadamias, roasted or dry roasted	5 nuts or $\frac{1}{2}$ tablespoon
Mixed nuts, dry or oil roasted	2 tablespoons
Peanut butter	1 flat tablespoon
Peanut butter, reduced fat	1 flat tablespoon
Peanuts, dry or oil roasted	20 nuts or 2 tablespoons
Pecans, dry or oil roasted	7 halves or 2 tablespoons
Pine nuts, dried	2 tablespoons
Pistachios, dry roasted	$2\frac{1}{2}$ tablespoons
Pumpkin kernels, dried	2 tablespoons
Sesame seeds	2 tablespoons
Sunflower seeds, dry or oil roasted	2 tablespoons
Tahini (sesame butter)	1 flat tablespoon
Walnuts, black, chopped	2 tablespoons
Walnuts, English, chopped	8 nuts or 2 tablespoons

OILS

Canola	2 teaspoons
Corn	2 teaspoons
Olive	2 teaspoons
Peanut	2 teaspoons
Safflower	2 teaspoons
Soybean	2 teaspoons
Soybean/cottonseed	2 teaspoons
Sunflower	2 teaspoons

SALAD DRESSINGS/SANDWICH SPREADS

Save calories and a fat serving by using nonfat salad dressings and nonfat sandwich spreads. Be sure to use only 4 tablespoons so that you don't have to count it as a daily serving.

Blue cheese, low-calorie	6 flat tablespoons
French, low-calorie	6 flat tablespoons
Italian, low-calorie	12 tablespoons

Italian, regular	1 1/2 tablespoons
Mayonnaise, imitation, low-calorie	2 1/2 flat tablespoons
Mayonnaise, light	2 flat tablespoons
Mayonnaise, regular, low-calorie	2 1/2 flat tablespoons
Ranch, low-calorie	3 flat tablespoons
Tartar sauce, low-calorie	3 flat tablespoons
Thousand Island, low-calorie	4 flat tablespoons
Vinaigrette	1 1/4 tablespoons
Vinegar and oil	1 1/4 tablespoons
Hummus	3 flat tablespoons

VEGETABLES

Olives, all types	20

FAT "FOES"

FOOD   SERVING SIZE

BUTTER AND WHIPPED CREAM

Stick	1 flat tablespoon
Pat	2 1/2 pats
Whipped cream	2 tablespoons

COOKING FATS

Bacon fat	2 flat teaspoons
Beef fat	2 flat teaspoons
Chicken fat	2 flat teaspoons
Lard	2 flat teaspoons
Margarine (any type)	2 flat teaspoons
Vegetable shortening	2 flat teaspoons

NUTS

Coconut, shredded/grated	1/5 cup

SALAD DRESSINGS/SANDWICH SPREADS

Save calories and a fat serving by using nonfat salad dressings and nonfat sandwich spreads. If you limit these nonfat dressings to 4 tablespoons, you will still have a fat serving to spare.

Blue cheese, regular	1 1/2 flat tablespoons
Cream cheese	2 flat tablespoons
French, regular	1 1/2 flat tablespoons
Mayonnaise, regular	1 flat tablespoon
Miracle Whip	2 flat tablespoons
Ranch, regular	1 1/2 flat tablespoons
Tartar sauce, regular	1 flat tablespoon
Thousand Island, regular	1 1/2 flat tablespoons

As we mentioned in the previous chapter, keeping a food diary is essential to guarantee your success. Tracking what you eat holds you accountable for your actions, and you'll see all the steps you have taken to fire up your metabolism. On the following page is a sample food diary with serving sizes. Now that you know how to count each serving size, you can follow along.

If a food has fewer than ten calories per serving, you don't have to count the food into your servings for the day, but don't have more than four servings of any of these "free" foods daily. Such foods include balsamic vinegar, butter spray, some nonfat salad dressings, diet sodas, Crystal Light, sugar-free Jell-O, and many other sugar-free products. Be sure that you stick to the serving size listed. In addition, if you want a serving of a food that is not on our lists that is twenty to twenty-five calories a serving, such as low-sugar jelly, sugar-free syrup, light syrup, or some nonfat salad dressings, simply count one serving as two of your four "free" foods.

Sample Food Diary

DAY, TIME	FOOD	SERVING SIZE	TOTAL SERVINGS
	Includes condiments, butter, dressings, drinks	*tablespoon, cup, ounce, etc.*	*You will learn how many carb, protein, and fat servings you need to fire up your metabolism as you read chapters 3, 4, and 5.*
Monday 8:30 A.M. (just woke up)	Raisin Bran	½ cup	1 "always" carb
	Nonfat (skim) milk	¾ cup	1 "thumbs-up" protein
	Water	2 cups	2 waters
11 A.M. (at office)	Nonfat, light yogurt	4 ounces	½ "thumbs-up" protein
	Low-fat, no-sugar-added granola	¼ cup	1 "always" carb
9–12 A.M.	Water	2 cups	2 waters
1:15 P.M.	Mexican wrap:		
	Small whole wheat wrap	1 wrap	1 "always" carb
	Chicken breast	size of 3 middle fingers	1 "thumbs-up" protein
	cooked with cooking spray (Pam)	a spray	free
	Bell pepper, cooked	½ cup	1 veggie
	Onion, cooked	¼ cup	½ veggie
	Squash, cooked	½ cup	1 veggie
	Cheese, low-fat (mixed in wrap)	⅓ ounce (2 tsp.)	½ "thumbs-up" protein
	Cantaloupe, cubed	1 cup	1 fruit
	Water	1 cup	1 water
4:15 P.M. (snack, at office)	Red and green bell pepper strips	½ cup	1 veggie
	Hummus	1½ flat tbsp.	½ "friendly" fat

6:00 P.M. (at office, about to go to dinner with coworkers)	Water	1 cup	1 water
	Hot tea	1 cup	Free
7:15 P.M. (at restaurant)	Mixed green dinner salad with cherry tomatoes and carrots	about 2 cups	2 veggies
	Balsamic vinegar	3 tbsp.	free
	Grilled swordfish steak (save extras for tomorrow's lunch)	4 ounces	2 "thumbs-up" proteins
	Brown rice	1 cup	2 "always" carbs
	Carrots, zucchini, and yellow squash, steamed	1 cup	2 veggies
8:30 P.M. (at home)	Water	2 cups	2 waters
	Strawberries	1/2 cup	1 fruit

TOTAL CARBS

Grain servings I need to fire it up: 5   # of grains I ate: 5 "always" carbs

Fruit servings I need to fire it up: 2   # of fruits I ate: 2

Vegetable servings I need to fire it up: at least 5   # of veggies I ate: 7 1/2

TOTAL PROTEIN

Protein servings I need to fire it up: 5   # of proteins I ate: 5

TOTAL FAT

Fat servings I need to fire it up: 1/2   # of fats I ate: 1/2

TOTAL WATER

Cups of water I need to fire up my metabolism: at least 8   # of cups of water I drank: 8

THREE

Choosing Carbohydrates Carefully

Myth Busters

MYTH: Vegetables are boring.

BUSTED: Vegetables roasted with your favorite spices are *not* boring. Try hot pepper, garlic, or onion. See page 67 for a list of ways to spice up your veggies.

MYTH: You can't sink your teeth into veggies.

BUSTED: Try filling up on a box of frozen spinach cooked with tomato sauce and sprinkled with Parmesan cheese.

MYTH: You can't enjoy vegetables without fattening dressings.

BUSTED: Try dipping your veggies in balsamic vinegar, salsa, barbecue sauce, nonfat yogurt and onion dip mix, or nonfat dressing.

MYTH: Carbohydrates are fattening.

BUSTED: Carbohydrates are not fattening. However, they do invite fattening toppings like butter, cream sauces, and sour cream, which lead to excess pounds. And people tend to overeat carbs; overeating anything causes weight gain.

MYTH: Eating bread and pasta isn't healthy.

BUSTED: Whole wheat pastas and whole wheat breads are extremely healthy and important for a speedy metabolism.

MYTH: You should eat carbohydrates only early in the day.

BUSTED: You need to eat *some* carbohydrates at every meal; they provide your body with energy and they are your body's fuel.

Our Twin Trial

in which we prove that carbohydrates are essential for keeping your metabolism sped up

We are both extremely energetic, and we owe much of our energy to eating plenty of "always" carbohydrates. We hypothesized that the guinea pig who would have to practically give up these carbohydrates would most likely be a "tired twin" during the course of the experiment.

As you can imagine, convincing Tammy that it was her turn to be the nutritional science experiment took a little more than just Lyssie's reminder that her past guinea pig experience resulted in salvaging her hair. So Lyssie also tried to work her seventeen-minute age seniority to her advantage, but Tammy wouldn't budge.

To be fair, we flipped a coin and let that dictate our nutritional fate for this experiment and for the rest of our twin trials. As luck would have it, Lyssie lost. This meant that she was doomed to give up her body's most efficient metabolism-revving fuel and her body's best source of energy, the "always" carbohydrates. Instead, she would be forced to fuel her body, as most Americans do, primarily with "sometimes" and "rarely" carbohydrates. Although all carbohydrates, including the "sometimes" and "rarely" ones, provide energy for the body, it's only the "always" carbohydrates that kick the metabolism into high gear.

Lyssie: I knew the severity of the results: I had witnessed countless clients who initially came to us loading up their bodies primarily with "sometimes" and "rarely" carbohydrates and experienced energy highs and crashes, food cravings and frequent hunger, and a body fat count that was through the roof. After making changes in their diets so that they were eating mostly "always" carbohydrates, our clients rarely experienced hunger pangs, had few if any food cravings, had more energy than ever, and most of all, their metabolism had sped up, causing them to lose innumerable pounds.

Now it was my turn to prove just how damaging overeating "sometimes" and "rarely" carbohydrates can be. Would someone like myself, with tons of energy and substantial amounts of dietary discipline, succumb to the ill effects of eating mainly "sometimes" and "rarely" carbohydrates? Would I have energy crashes and food cravings and a slow metabolism that would lead to fat gain? I feared the worst and complained for an entire hour after losing the flip—and that was even before the trial began. Being forced to eat the "sometimes" and "rarely" carbohydrates is worth making a fuss over.

So for four weeks we both had our usual daily eight carbohydrate servings. Only now I met my carbohydrate requirements by having five servings of "sometimes" carbohydrates and three servings of "rarely" carbohydrates rather than the primarily "always" carbohydrates I usually ate.

The changes started in the morning. Instead of eating my usual breakfast of homemade granola (our mom makes this herself with whole oats—"always" carb—soy flour, and nuts and no hydrogenated oils, and sends it to me), I chose a "sometimes" breakfast cereal, Special K, and ate that with my usual soy milk and an apple. By midmorning, I was already sliding on the slippery slope of carbs. I was hungry before lunch for the first time in years, and I was craving more food so that I could have my usual energy.

Most mornings I eat breakfast and then go to the gym. My breakfast gives me fuel for my workout and tides me over until about 9:00 or 9:30 when I have my midmorning snack. However, after having Special K, I was hungry in the middle of my aerobic exercise. Not surprisingly, exhaustion followed hunger, and before I knew it my usual pace on the treadmill slowed. When I switched to the bike, I was completely zonked.

So much for burning calories that morning. All I wanted was my midmorning snack. I was ravenous. My usual postworkout yogurt didn't make a dent in my hunger! I felt like I needed more food, which I didn't want to have, because the extra food would compromise the trial.

Thinking that the Special K might be to blame, in the next days I experimented with several different "sometimes" carbohydrates to see which would make me feel the best. I tried Honey Nut Cheerios, Chex, Product 19, white toast, and Cream of Wheat. Eventually, I wound up choosing a plain, white English muffin with soy milk and an apple, as this seemed to be the most satiating and energizing, yet it too still left my stomach rumbling.

One week into the trial, I got to the point where I couldn't take it any longer. I cheated and gave in to my temptation. I started with a post-yogurt pretzel. Later in the month, that turned into two or three.

I really tried to make this experiment as painless as possible by simply eating the same main meals I usually ate, only replacing "always" carbohydrates with the "sometimes" and "rarely" ones. Now I had my regular sandwich on white bread. At dinner, I replaced brown rice, whole wheat pita, and whole wheat tortillas with their refined counterparts—white rice, white pita, and white flour tortillas.

Overall, besides making several taste adjustments, the main effects that I experienced from my carb switch were that hunger came on shortly after meals and I felt less energetic. I was most affected after breakfast, when the "sometimes" carbohydrate was quickly burned because I didn't have a whole lot of fiber or protein or fat with the meal to slow the digestion and to keep delivering energy to me.

After four weeks of this experiment, my body fat had gone up 3½ percent.

I was shocked. The only change I made was in the *type* of carbs I ate. My serving portions and frequencies were the same, and although my lunches varied among tuna, turkey, and peanut butter sandwiches, they were always on white English muffins or white pita. For dinner I had fish, chicken, turkey, or veggie burgers, but white rice, white pasta, or white bread and white buns always accompanied them. My snacks of low-fat cheese and whole wheat crackers were made on saltines or Wheat Thins. So, although a 3½ percent change in body fat may not sound like much, it is significant when you consider that my exercise routine and most of my other food choices remained the same.

The psychological consequences of the weight gain were *much* worse than the physical. The Saturday night before this trial ended, I went to a wedding, which I had been eagerly anticipating for months. I had bought the *perfect,* sleek, beautiful black dress, and I couldn't wait to wear it when I saw my old friends. One problem: The dress no longer looked quite so perfect. It was snug and unflattering. I did the only decent thing I could while attempting to save my pride. I grabbed my biggest Pashmina and draped it over the dress. It might as well have been a curtain—it was so big that it covered everything from my shoulders to my knees (thank God something fit perfectly!).

The good news is that I had another wedding a couple of months

We used body fat percentage as a means to measure the results of our trials. Your body fat percentage is the percent of your total body weight that comes from fat. We did not use the scale to measure our results—weight alone is not a clear indicator of how much body fat you have gained or lost because it does not distinguish between pounds that come from body fat and those that come from lean body mass or muscle. To get an idea of how the scale is much less important than body fat percentage, consider this: A five-foot-ten bodybuilder who weighs 225 pounds and is extremely lean has a very low body fat of 6 percent yet seems overweight if you just look at the scale. On the other hand, a five-foot-ten potbellied, squishy man who appears to have no muscle may weigh only two-thirds of the bodybuilder's weight yet have more than twice as much fat on him, at around 22 percent.

If a two hundred-pound man increases his body fat by 2 percent, he will have gained four pounds of body fat. If a one hundred-pound woman increases her body fat by 2 percent, she will have gained two pounds.

later, and now I had real inspiration to keep clear of "sometimes" and "rarely" carbs again—I wanted to look good in that dress! Choosing the wrong carbohydrates, such as I was forced to do, is an error that most Americans make unwittingly.

How Does Nixing Carbohydrates Cause My Body to Lose Muscle?

Muscles, like movement, burn calories. And carbohydrates, not just protein, play an important role in maintaining your muscles. So without carbohydrates, your body loses muscle. Without muscle, you cannot burn calories.

If you don't give your body carbohydrates, the fuel it needs for your brain, red blood cells, central nervous system, and muscles, your body will feel threatened and will be forced to use an alternative fuel to provide energy—protein. The protein you eat will be converted into glucose (fuel) and, in addition, just a little fat will be used for energy. Counting on protein for energy diverts it from its main job, repairing your muscles and tissues and boosting your immune system. So without carbohydrates you won't be able to build muscle efficiently, because your body will turn to the protein to carry on other more immediate body functions.

That's trouble. Having lean muscle mass is one of the most important components of a fired-up metabolism. *The more muscle you have, the more calories your body burns* (see Chapter 11). So clearly, if your body can't build or repair muscle (and muscle degrades daily and relies on protein to help to rebuild it), you will have less muscle and will burn fewer calories than you did when you had more muscle. What could be more counterproductive?

If Carbohydrates Are Needed to Fire Up My Metabolism and to Prevent My Body from Losing Muscle, Why Do People Lose Weight When They Cut Out Carbohydrates?

Without carbohydrates you may lose weight *at first*. Low-carb, high-protein, low-calorie eating plans (such as the Atkins diet, which encourages you to load up on high-protein foods like meats but does not include most carbohydrates) cause you to lose a lot of water. Here's why: When your body digests protein, it breaks it down into urea, a toxin that needs to be flushed out of your body. Your body relies on its water stores to flush these toxins out with your urine.

Although this is a normal and healthy response to eating protein, this means that when your diet is high in protein, you draw on a large amount of your body's water stores to flush out these toxins. Considering that your body weight is at least 60 percent water, you have a substantial amount of water weight that can be lost immediately. What's more, you store carbohydrates in your muscles as energy (glycogen). For every pound of muscle glycogen, you store three pounds of water. So without carbohydrates for muscle energy, you won't have that water in your body either.

But water loss is not fat loss; water weight loss is only a quick fix when you are paying attention to the scale, as it can be gained back in *minutes* after drinking or eating.

Next, you now know that if you don't have carbohydrates, your body loses muscle, and this creates a weight loss too. (Consuming protein will help you to rebuild some muscle; however, you will not be able to rebuild your muscle at the rate at which you are losing it.) Muscle weighs a lot more than fat, which is one of the main reasons that you lose weight.

Weight loss does not necessarily equal fat loss. If you lose water and muscle, you may be a lot lighter on the scale, but you will still look and feel flabby. So remember, replacing carbohydrates with protein gets you only water and muscle loss.

Skimping on Carbs Slows Your Metabolism— That's Why Low-Carb Fad Diets Don't Deliver Lasting Results

Have you ever wondered why after you successfully lost weight on a very low-carbohydrate diet you gained it all back as soon as you started eating normally? As you now know, part of this regained weight is due to the water weight that you initially lost.

Another reason for the rebound is that you slowed your metabolism by avoiding carbohydrates. As we mentioned, if you don't eat carbohydrates, your body will feel threatened and will turn to an alternative fuel—protein. Since protein is not designed to provide your body with energy, if your body is forced to try to make energy from it, you feel exhausted. This means that if you want to have any energy, feeding yourself carbohydrates is essential. And when it comes to the speed of your metabolism, you better believe that you want energy. Remember, all movements burn calories, so if you are exhausted and don't have energy to move, you will slow your metabolism. That's why people who try to avoid carbohydrates yet load up on meat and eggs or carbohydrate-free protein shakes feel tired; they are not giving their body the energy it needs, and they will never be able to fire up their metabolism to their maximum potential. And that is why they may never obtain their long-term weight-loss goals. Without carbohydrates they don't feel good enough or have enough energy to achieve their goals.

Carb Depletion Depresses Your Metabolic Rate

As if this weren't bad enough, when you skimp on carbohydrates, your body cannot completely burn fat.

Any registered dietitian will tell you that body fat burns in the fire of carbohydrates. That's right: If you want to burn fat, you need carbohydrates. For fat to be completely dismantled and metabolized, carbohydrate molecules must bond with fat molecules. Without the carbohydrate, fat fragments have no choice but to combine with each other, forming ketone bodies—the end product of incomplete fat breakdown.

Ketones then become an alternative brain fuel, and this can be dangerous because ketones throw off your body's acid-base balance, causing a condition called ketosis. Ketones are acidic, and when their concentration rises in your body, as it does when you follow any very low-carbohydrate diet such as the Atkins diet, there are consequences. Potential long-term complications include heart disease, bone loss, and kidney damage. The amount of ketone bodies you make depends on how much glucose (carbohydrates) is available to your system—without carbohydrates, you make a lot of ketones. Although there are long-term consequences, most people probably can't stay on the diet long enough to experience them. Most respond almost immediately in the short term, experiencing headaches, sleepiness, lack of energy, nausea, dehydration, and diarrhea. Who can have energy to burn calories while experiencing these symptoms? Most people would be lucky to muster together enough energy to get out of bed. In addition, many people are embarrassed to go out in public, as ketones cause *very* bad breath. Worse yet, when ketosis sets in, it is the signal that muscle tissue wasting has begun and the metabolism is being slowed. Remember, the more muscle you have, the faster your metabolism. Again, this is a double whammy: Your body is burning up its muscle for energy, thereby burning less fat and fewer calories, and any fat that your body does burn is only partially burned.

Carbohydrates: You Know You Need Them, Now It's Time to Learn *How* to Eat Them

We have been doing it all wrong. We choose the wrong carbohydrates ("sometimes" and "rarely" carbs), and then we make these troublesome carbs worse. The following mistakes demonstrate how you may easily fall into the traps.

Mistake #1: We don't leave our carbs alone. We slather them with calorie-dense fatty spreads and toppings.

For instance, you might feel virtuous for choosing a bagel over a Pop Tart, but most people don't eat their bagel dry—they add butter or cream cheese, which are pure fat. Baked potatoes usually get butter or sour cream, and pasta is always accompanied by sauce.

Although it is good to eat a carbohydrate with a little bit of protein and/or fat, fat servings add up so quickly that if you don't know the appropriate size of a serving, you will inevitably eat too much and gain weight. For example, a slice of bread, which is equal in calories to an apple, suddenly has the same amount of calories as a McDonald's hamburger when you spread just several teaspoons of butter on it. And if you top a ninety-calorie baked potato with just a half cup of sour cream and a couple of teaspoons of butter, you might as well eat a McDonald's quarter-pounder with cheese—it would be equal in calories. Similarly, a two-hundred-calorie portion of pasta suddenly becomes five hundred calories when it is in an Alfredo, vodka, or oil sauce.

So it's no wonder that we are gaining weight from carbohydrates. But the whole food group shouldn't suffer.

If you choose the right ones—and avoid adding fat to them—carbs will be your best friend in the quest to fire up your metabolism.

TIPS

MULLING OVER WHICH MUFFIN TO CHOOSE? DON'T CHOOSE ANY—EVEN IF IT'S BRAN OR OAT—UNLESS YOU'RE LOOKING TO MUFF UP THAT METABOLISM. Most muffins are packed with fat and sugar and lead to weight gain when eaten too frequently.

POP TART? DON'T EVEN THINK ABOUT PUTTING THAT IN YOUR CART! Two hundred calories of fat and sugar. Need we say more?

AVOID AUNTIE ANNE'S PRETZELS. SHE'S NOT QUITE THE WHOLE-SOME AUNT SHE SEEMS TO BE. At 350 calories for a pretzel *without* butter, and 450 calories with butter, this carbohydrate will overwhelm your metabolism.

ZUCCHINI BREAD . . . CARROT CAKE . . . BANANA MUFFINS. DON'T BE FOOLED. These are high-calorie, high-fat "rarely" desserts, not vegetables.

IS THAT A HASH BROWN? YOU BETTER GET OUT OF TOWN! These oven-fried potatoes will fire up your metabolism. Peel and shred two large boiled potatoes. Mix in 2 tablespoons finely chopped onion, 1 minced clove of garlic, $1/2$ teaspoon fresh thyme (or $1/4$ teaspoon dried thyme), and $1/8$ teaspoon pepper. Spray a ten-inch nonstick skillet with vegetable cooking spray and heat until hot over medium heat. Add the potato mixture and cook until browned on both sides, flipping once, six to seven minutes total. Makes four servings. Each serving equals one "always" carbohydrate.

Mistake #2: Portion sizes far exceed recommendations. The American Dietetic Association recommends that you consume six to eleven servings per day from the grain (carbohydrate) group. This means that a small woman should consume about six servings per day, whereas a larger or more active woman or a smaller man should consume about eight servings. A larger, more active man should consume about eleven servings.

But most people don't know what these serving sizes look like. Take, for example, Marge, our typical fairly inactive client who comes to our office wanting to lose weight. We tell Marge that she should be consuming six servings from the grain group per day. Marge is shocked and replies in horror, "I could never eat that much without gaining weight!" She tells us that the only foods she eats from the grain group is her morning bagel and her pasta at dinner and she cannot possibly eat more without gaining weight. However, after asking Marge a few questions about the bagel and the pasta, we discover that she definitely is not consuming her goal of six servings from the grain group per day; Marge is actually consuming a whopping eleven servings. Her New York deli bagel is actually equal to five servings from the grain group, and her seemingly small pasta dinner is equal to six servings.

How could this be? Here's how. One-half of a small prepackaged bagel (about 3½" diameter, the size of hockey puck) is considered one grain serving. So one small bagel is two servings. And ½ cup (½ cup would fit in your hand) of cooked rice, cooked cereal, or cooked pasta is also considered one serving. So Marge's large bagel (2½ times the size of a small, prepackaged bagel), combined with her three cups of pasta for dinner sends her soaring to eleven grain servings—the amount that a large, active male would need, not Marge, who is smaller and fairly inactive, and wants to lose weight. Later, as Marge realizes that the cause of her weight gain is her large portion sizes, she embarrassedly admits to us that she forgot to mention that she has been adding croutons to her salad at lunch. "Should I count the croutons toward the grain group, as well?" Yes, Marge, you should.

As you now know, Marge's large portion sizes were causing her to gain weight and contributing to the misconception that carbohydrates are fattening. You may have also realized that Marge was making another common carbohydrate mistake. She chose the quickly digested, refined "sometimes" and "rarely" carbohydrates. (If you did notice this mistake, you are learning how to spot the carbohydrates you should limit.) To make sure that you don't overeat carbs, as Marge did, see pages 65 to 66 to learn the Rule of Hand for grains. Just keep in mind that the right carbohydrates *must* be included in your diet if you want to fire up your metabolism and lose weight.

Also keep in mind that when you eat too many calories, even

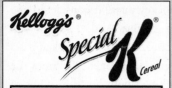

Nutrition Facts

Serving Size 1 Cup (31g/1.1 oz.)
Servings per Package About 6

Amount Per Serving	Cereal	Cereal with 1/2 Cup Vitamins A&D Fat Free Milk
Calories	110	150
Calories from Fat	0	0

	% Daily Value**	
Total Fat 0g*	0%	0%
Saturated Fat 0g	0%	0%
Cholesterol 0mg	0%	0%
Sodium 220mg	9%	12%
Potassium 60mg	2%	7%
Total Carbohydrate 22g	7%	9%
Dietary Fiber less than 1g	3%	3%
Sugars 4g		
Other Carbohydrate 18g		
Protein 7g	3%	13%
Vitamin A	15%	20%
Vitamin C	35%	35%
Calcium	0%	15%
Iron	45%	45%
Vitamin E	35%	35%
Thiamin	35%	40%
Riboflavin	35%	45%
Niacin	35%	35%
Vitamin B$_6$	100%	100%
Folic Acid	100%	100%
Vitamin B$_{12}$	100%	110%
Phosphorus	6%	20%
Magnesium	4%	8%
Zinc	6%	8%
Selenium	10%	10%

* Amount in cereal. One half cup of fat free milk contributes an additional 40 calories, 65mg sodium, 6g total carbohydrate (6g sugars), and 4g protein.

** Percent Daily Values are based on a 2,000 calorie diet. Your daily values may be higher or lower depending on your calorie needs:

		Calories	2,000	2,500
Total Fat	Less than		65g	80g
Sat. Fat	Less than		20g	25g
Cholesterol	Less than		300mg	300mg
Sodium	Less than		2,400mg	2,400mg
Potassium			3,500mg	3,500mg
Total Carbohydrate			300g	375g
Dietary Fiber			25g	30g
Protein			50g	65g

Calories per gram: Fat 9 • Carbohydrate 4 • Protein 4

Ingredients: Rice, wheat gluten, sugar, defatted wheat germ, salt, high fructose corn syrup, dried whey, malt flavoring, calcium caseinate, **Vitamins and Minerals:** ascorbic acid (vitamin C), alpha tocopherol acetate (vitamin E), reduced iron, niacinamide, pyridoxine hydrochloride (vitamin B$_6$), riboflavin (vitamin B$_2$), thiamin hydrochloride (vitamin B$_1$), vitamin A palmitate, folic acid and vitamin B$_{12}$. To maintain quality, BHT has been added to the packaging.

CONTAINS WHEAT AND MILK INGREDIENTS.

As you can see, the main ingredient in the cereal is rice—white, refined rice. If the cereal were made from brown, unrefined rice, it would specify "brown" rice, and the cereal would contain more fiber. However, each cup of Special K has less than one gram of fiber. This is not enough to make the energy boost from the carbohydrates long-lasting; you will soon need more energy, and you will also be hungry, as there is no fiber to slow digestion. Alas, Special K doesn't qualify as an "always" carbohydrate.

when your metabolism is moving in high gear, it is still possible to overdo it. We refer to this as "overwhelming your metabolism." An extreme example is a small female who ate two cheeseburgers and three pieces of pie for dinner. Her metabolism would be overwhelmed by so much food and wouldn't be able to burn off all of the calories, so her body would be forced to store some of them as fat.

Mistake #3: We choose the wrong carbs. Granted, most people know that a bag of french fries is not a healthful choice. But there is still a lot of confusion about what is and isn't healthy. For example, you might choose a "sometimes" cereal, such as Special K, for breakfast, thinking that you are making a healthy choice. But in reality, such a cereal is a very distant cousin of the original grain that grew from the ground. This processed breakfast cereal is not a wholesome fruit, vegetable, or grain; it is *not* the carbohydrate we like, such as Raisin Bran or oatmeal, where the bran and oats are in their natural form. The more processed the food, the more susceptible you are to energy highs and crashes, which cause you to reach for yet more food for a boost.

What Makes the "Sometimes" and "Rarely" Carbohydrates so Bad?

Your muscles can store carbs, unlike protein and fats, as energy. However, even though the "sometimes" and "rarely" carbohydrates provide an immediate source of energy, it's not long-lasting energy. You might think of them as one-night stands: satisfying for the moment, but empty in the long run.

When manufacturers want to make white bread or white rice, they "refine" or "process" the carbohydrate, remove its bran and germ (fiber and nutrients)—leaving just the endosperm (starch).

Because there's no fiber in these carbs to slow digestion, you get hungry again within an hour. You see, without fiber, glucose (fuel) quickly enters your bloodstream, causing your blood sugar to skyrocket. The next thing you know, your body responds by releasing a

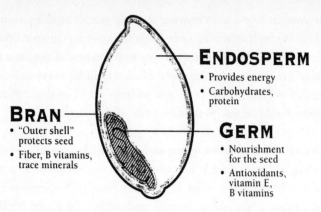

ENDOSPERM
- Provides energy
- Carbohydrates, protein

BRAN
- "Outer shell" protects seed
- Fiber, B vitamins, trace minerals

GERM
- Nourishment for the seed
- Antioxidants, vitamin E, B vitamins

Reprinted with permission of General Mills, Inc., from *Go With the Grain Educational Resource Kit*.

surge of insulin, which shuttles glucose out of the blood and into the cells for energy.

However, due to the large quantity of insulin you've just secreted, the glucose in the blood is quickly removed. The brain receives the signal that it needs more fuel, and the next thing you know, you are reaching for more food to provide your body with more energy. In reality, your body should not need fuel, as it received food an hour or so ago. Consequently, you end up consuming excess calories.

TIPS

THROW AWAY YOUR CRISPIX, RICE KRISPIES, CORN FLAKES, AND RICE CHEX! Cereals like these are made from refined grain and lack fiber. Keep in mind that a "sometimes" cereal, like any of these, is always a better choice than a "rarely" cereal that has a lot of added sugar or fat, like Corn Pops or Post Selects Blueberry Morning. If you choose to eat a "rarely" cereal, have only one serving—and remember that, depending on the cereal, a serving is sometimes just ½ cup, not necessarily a full bowl. And then instead of allowing yourself a "sometimes" carbohydrate two times out of ten, permit yourself only one serving out of ten.

NIX SODA—UNLESS YOU'RE LOOKING TO CRASH. The sugary boost of sodas gives you a blood sugar high—and then a low. Even though your body has received calories, you end up craving food and then overeating. Diet soda is okay but not as good as water.

JUST BECAUSE BROWN SUGAR LOOKS MORE NATURAL DOESN'T MEAN IT'S BETTER THAN WHITE SUGAR. Sugar is sugar. Brown or white, it's all the same—a source of calories with no valuable nutrients.

SHUNNING PASTA, MACARONI, AND RIGATONI? THAT'S BALONEY—AS LONG AS YOU LIMIT YOURSELF TO A FIST-SIZE PORTION A DAY! Remember, white pasta is a "sometimes" carbohydrate, so you should eat it only two out of every ten times that you have a grain, and be sure to limit it to a maximum of a fist-size portion every day. Depending on your fist size, this will give you two or three of your grain servings for the day. Then fill your stomach with veggies that are mixed in the sauce and include the appropriate portion size of protein (see Chapter 2). If you prepare the whole wheat pasta yourself, still limit it to just the size of your fist. A bonus: You will have a "sometimes" carbohydrate to spare.

The unprocessed "always" carbohydrates also keep their bran—the part that contains fiber. Fiber has many benefits: It slows digestion, causing the carbohydrate to be released gradually into your bloodstream, thereby providing a more ongoing, long-lasting release of energy, rather than a quick burst. Therefore, fiber helps keep your energy levels even, enabling you to be active all day long and burn more calories through activity. (To understand why having energy to perform more activity is critical for firing up your metabolism, see Chapter 10.)

Fiber helps your metabolic rate stay revved longer. Thanks to a process called diet-induced thermogenesis, when you eat, your body has to work to digest, absorb, transport, metabolize, and process nutrients. This causes the muscles in your gastrointestinal tract to speed up their rhythmic contractions, and this increase in the body's activity produces heat, causing you to burn a few more calories. Because fiber slows and steadies digestion, when you eat an "always" carbohydrate, which is a good source of fiber, you benefit from calorie-burning thermogenesis for longer.

TIPS

WHEN IT COMES TO RAISIN BRAN, BE A FAN! This cereal is made from the whole grain, whose nutrients help turn your food into usable energy. Raisin Bran is also packed with fiber, which helps you to have a sustained release of energy. Your blood sugar rises gradually and remains stable without crashing. This is great news—you don't feel the urgent need for more fuel. "Two scoops" of Raisin Bran (one cup of this particular cereal) are equal to two grain servings.

TOSS THAT SEVEN-GRAIN AND NINE-GRAIN BREAD. They may look healthy, but seven-grain and nine-grain bread are not made from whole grains. Rather, they are composed of refined flour. The dough is sprinkled with other grains but not enough to make the slightest difference and certainly not enough to add a decent amount of fiber and to keep the metabolic boost of the carbohydrates lasting longer. Check the ingredient label of your bread. If the first grain doesn't say "whole" before it, stay away.

A TOAST TO FRENCH TOAST. But only if it is cooked right, by dipping whole wheat bread in egg or Egg Beaters and skim milk and then frying it in only cooking spray. If you must use syrup, use a "light" syrup and limit to 2 tablespoons. Better yet, top with fresh or frozen fruit. This adds fiber instead of sugar, keeping your energy level stable after the meal.

MOVIE POPCORN WILL PLAY YOU. Popcorn at theaters has enough fat to flub up your metabolism. Instead, try air-popped popcorn (make it at home) without added oil. This "always" carbohydrate is only one hundred calories for three cups!

WANNA CRACKER? TRY AK-MAK, WASA, OR RY-KRISP WHOLE-GRAIN. These choices have even more fiber than whole wheat bread and are low in fat, calories, and sodium. What a way to add a crunch to a salad without croutons. Run the cracker under water for a second, then microwave in a microwave-safe, resealable plastic bag for about twenty seconds, and you will have a soft, nutrient-packed, low-calorie bread that can replace higher-calorie, lower-fiber breads. It is sure to fire you up.

SWITCH FROM WHITE BREAD TO WHOLE WHEAT. Just this one change alone may provide you with up to two grams more fiber per slice. Not to mention that you will have a "sometimes" carbohydrate to spare!

BAGEL BUST! UNLESS YOU SCOOP THE INSIDE OUT. Most deli bagels contain $3\frac{1}{2}$ to 6 of your carbohydrate servings. And the supposed "whole wheat" bagels are only sprinkled with whole wheat flour—the rest is mostly refined flour. So if you must eat it, take its insides out. Or if you choose not to scoop, keep it to once a week and eat only half of it.

MAKING OR ORDERING A PIZZA? USE WHOLE WHEAT DOUGH. Skip the refined white dough if you want to skip out of a possibly slowed metabolism. The energy and metabolic boost of the carbohydrates from white dough drop much sooner than from whole wheat dough.

WHAT A WAFFLE! (THAT IS, IF IT IS WHOLE WHEAT.) Yes, these do exist! Just check the ingredients label on waffle packages to find the brand that says "whole" before the grain. Or on a weekend, when you have more time, use a waffle iron and prepare it with whole wheat flour. If you want a lighter, fluffier waffle, use whole wheat pastry flour.

SUSHI CAN BE SUPER . . . IF YOU ORDER IT MADE WITH BROWN RICE. Ask your server if your sushi can come with brown rice. Why not feel more satiated and get some extra fiber while revving your metabolism? If you can't get sushi with brown rice, order sashimi with a side of brown rice. If the restaurant doesn't have brown rice, you may have to settle for white rice and use your "sometimes" carbs for the day.

The list below clarifies serving sizes. Then follow the steps on pages 63 to 65 and see the Daily Grain Servings table to find out how many servings someone of your size and level of activity needs.

One serving from the carbohydrate/grain group is equal to:

- ½ hamburger bun or ½ English muffin

- 1 slice of bread

- 1 small (2 ounces) roll, muffin, or biscuit

- 1 ounce (½ cup) ready-to-eat cereal

- ½ cup cooked cereal, rice, or pasta

- 3–4 small or 2 large crackers

See pages 23 to 31 for the complete lists of "always," "sometimes," and "rarely" carbohydrates.

Rule of Hand for grains:

- A small woman's fist = 1 cup of pasta, rice, or cooked cereal (two servings of a grain carbohydrate)

- A man's fist = 1½ cups pasta, rice, or cooked cereal (three servings of a grain carbohydrate)

- Food that fits in the cup of your hand = ½ cup (one serving when it comes to pasta, rice, or cooked cereal)

The Fire Up Your Metabolism Plan: Put Your Metabolism in High Gear

To follow the Fire Up Your Metabolism plan to burn away body fat and jump-start your metabolism, first figure out what your body *needs* by following these steps.

STEP 1

You are fairly sedentary: You exercise once or twice a week. Multiply your weight in pounds by 10.

Your weight in pounds ____ × 10 = ____ (Use this number for Step 2.)

If you are more than twenty pounds overweight, or if you would like to see faster results, multiply your weight by 9.5.

Your weight in pounds ____ × 9.5 = ____ (Use this number for Step 2.)

You are moderately active: You perform cardiovascular exercise at least three to four times a week for at least twenty to thirty minutes, and you lift weights several times a week, or you have a job that requires lifting and manual labor, or you are an active mom who is always lifting your kids and groceries. Multiply your weight in pounds by 11.

Your weight in pounds ____ × 11 = ____ (Use this number for Step 2.)

If you are more than twenty pounds overweight, or if you want to see faster results, multiply your weight by 10.

Your weight in pounds ____ × 10 = ____ (Use this number for Step 2.)

You exercise fairly intensely: You do cardiovascular exercise at least five times a week for at least thirty minutes, and you lift weights fairly intensely several times per week. Multiply your weight by 12.

Your weight in pounds ____ × 12 = _____ (Use this number for Step 2.)

If you are more than 20 pounds overweight, or if you want to see faster results, multiply your weight by 11.

Your weight in pounds ____ × 11 = _____ (Use this number for Step 2.)

You perform strenuous exercise: You do cardiovascular exercise *at least* five to six times a week for sixty minutes, and you lift weights rigorously *at least* three times per week. Multiply your weight by 13.

Your weight in pounds ____ × 13 = _____ (Use this number for Step 2.)

If you are more than 20 pounds overweight, or if you want to see faster results, multiply your weight times 12.

Your weight in pounds ____ × 12 = _____ (Use this number for Step 2.)

If your activity level falls between two categories, multiply your weight by the lower number and one half.

Example: Peter exercises cardiovascularly at least three to four times a week, and he lifts weights half of those times. This places him in the moderately active category. He should multiply his weight by 12. However, Peter performs the cardiovascular exercise for only about fifteen to twenty minutes per session, which is less than the twenty- to thirty-minute requirement for the moderately active category. Therefore, Peter should multiply his weight by 11.5.

Example: Claudia exercises cardiovascularly five times a week for at least thirty minutes, which places her in the fairly intense exercise category. However, Claudia lifts weights once a week at most. Instead of multiplying her weight by 13, as required for those in the fairly intense group, she falls between a factor of 12 and 13. Therefore, she should multiply by 12.5.

If you are overweight and you perform very little or no exercise, assume that you should have five grain servings.

If you answered yes to more than ten questions on the "Do You Have a Slow Metabolism?" test (page 5), or if you feel that you have a very slow metabolism for other reasons such as you are very inactive, are going through menopause, or have been overweight all of your life, you may choose to decrease the number of servings of grains you need daily by one serving.

STEP 2

Find your number from Step 1 in the table below. This will tell you how many servings of grain (carbohydrates) you need each day.

Daily Grain Servings

YOUR NUMBER FROM STEP 1*	YOUR LEVEL (To be applied in later chapters)	YOUR DAILY GRAIN SERVINGS
1,200	12	5
1,300	13	5
1,400	14	5
1,500	15	5
1,600	16	6
1,700	17	6
1,800	18	6
1,900	19	7
2,000	20	7 1/2
2,100	21	8
2,200	22	8
2,300	23	8

(continued on next page)

Daily Grain Servings *(cont.)*

YOUR NUMBER FROM STEP 1 *	YOUR LEVEL (To be applied in later chapters)	YOUR DAILY GRAIN SERVINGS
2,400	24	9
2,500	25	10
2,600	26	10
2,700	27	11
2,800	28	11
2,900	29	11½
3,000–3,100	30	11½
3,200	31	11½
3,300–3,400	32	12
3,500	33	12

*If your number is less than 1,200, use 1,200.

If you feel extremely hungry, add a grain serving or follow the plan at the next higher number.

Vegetables: Your Metabolism-Saving Medicine

At the end of the meal, vegetables always seem to be sitting on the plate; they are the resisted food. And we understand this—it's the meat and potatoes, the items that you can really sink your teeth into, that we love the most because they are so satisfying. However, it's time to think of veggies as your metabolism-saving medicine.

Vegetables, which we consider "always" carbohydrates, should be a part of at least half of your meals and snacks. With the exception of peas, potatoes, and corn, which are more calorie dense, you can eat as many vegetables as you want. They are low-calorie, fiber filled, and nutrient packed.

Vegetables are particularly great before a meal, as their fiber will start to fill you up and help you to eat less of other foods. Now before you start complaining about their lack of flavor—and before you give

All vegetables are carbohydrates. And all of them are "always" carbohydrates. Just be sure to keep them lean by not seasoning them with butter, oil, or any other fat source.

in to the temptation to add butter, oil, dressing, or other fats—let us give you some ways to please your taste buds when eating vegetables—without hurting your metabolism.

Seasoning Vegetables Without Calories

VEGETABLE	SPICE IT UP WITH
Asparagus	Black pepper, garlic powder, lemon, nutmeg, vinegar
Broccoli	Basil, black pepper, garlic powder, lemon, onion, oregano
Brussels sprouts	Chestnut, lemon, marjoram, nutmeg, oregano, sage
Cabbage	Caraway, celery, or poppy seeds; dry mustard; green pepper; onion; oregano; pimiento; vinegar
Carrots	Black pepper, chives, cloves, garlic powder, ginger, lemon, marjoram, mint, thyme
Cauliflower	Basil, chives, lemon, nutmeg, paprika, parsley, rosemary
Collard, Kale, Mustard, or Turnip Greens	Garlic powder, lemon, onions, oregano, parsley, vinegar
Cucumbers	Basil, dill, lemon, oregano, vinegar
Eggplant	Basil, chives, garlic powder, lemon, onion, oregano, parsley, tarragon
Green beans	Basil, celery, dill, garlic powder, lemon, low-sodium bouillon powder, nutmeg, onions, pimiento
Okra	Bay leaf, black pepper, lemon, thyme
Onions	Garlic powder, green pepper, nutmeg, red pepper
Tomatoes	Basil, bay leaf, black pepper, celery, curry, dill, garlic powder, onion, oregano, sage, savory, thyme

BROCCOLI BY THE BARREL . . . THAT'S THE WAY YOU SHOULD EAT THIS WEIGHT-LOSS POWER PLANT! Raw broccoli provides just twenty-five calories per cup, which will fill you up. The fibrousness of this carbohydrate means that it is digested gradually, providing a consistent release of fuel so that you have plenty of energy to burn calories—and you can benefit from thermogenesis.

PASS THE PEAS, PLEASE! BUT ONLY ½ CUP. Packed with fiber, vitamins, and especially vitamin C, peas give you a metabolic boost. However, limit to just ½ cup, as they are not as low in calories as most other veggies.

CALLING CAULIFLOWER. Already touted as an anticarcinogen, cauliflower also helps to rev your metabolism, as its fiber extends the metabolic boost of the cauliflower's carbohydrates. Trick those family members who aren't fans of this veggie by pureeing it with mashed potatoes for a great texture. The family will get more fiber and vitamins with fewer calories, yet won't taste a difference.

GO FOR THE GOLD! For a change, instead of a baked potato, choose a sweet potato that is about the size of your fist. This veggie has more nutrients than its white cousin but just as much fiber to extend the metabolism boost of the carbohydrate. (White potatoes are okay if you eat the fibrous skin.) As a bonus, you get a burst of beta-carotene, a powerful antioxidant that may help your body to fight off diseases such as heart disease and cancer.

TOMATO SAUCE—NOT ONLY FOR PASTA! Tomato sauce is packed with nutrients and doesn't weigh you down like other fatty sauces. Use canned, crushed tomatoes (lots of fiber) and add garlic, oregano, and pepper to top different types of grains, such as barley, bulgur, couscous, or millet. Or top your baked potato with tomato sauce and pepper.

FORGET ABOUT THAT LETTUCE SALAD FOR LUNCH. Surprisingly, if your salad consists of lettuce topped mainly with vegetables, you aren't revving your metabolism the way you should be. First of all, the low-calorie veggies aren't providing enough calories to provide a significant source of energy. In addition, this only-carbohydrate meal won't keep you satiated for long, and within an hour or two you'll be ravenous and ready for more food. What's more, if you have added one scoop of full-fat dressing, you are getting five hundred extra calories that you didn't bargain for (causing you to gain one pound of weight a week). So if you want to stay lean and satiated, make sure to include in your vegetable salad a slightly more substantial "always" carbohydrate and a "thumbs-up" protein or a "friendly" fat.

Do be warned, canned vegetables are not quite as nutritious as frozen or fresh. Some of the water-soluble vitamins in canned vegetables leach out into the water they are packed in, and sodium is added in the canning process. However, eating canned vegetables is better than forgoing vegetables altogether. (If you do eat canned veggies, reduce the sodium by rinsing the veggies in a strainer under cold water.) When eating canned fruits, choose those that are canned in water or in their own juice rather than in syrup. Added syrup makes an "al-

---

Get more veggies without blinking an eye. You'll fill up faster, too.

- Order your pizzas stacked with vegetables and your pastas topped with mushrooms, broccoli, and other veggies.

- Stack your sandwiches with lettuce, tomatoes, and sprouts.

- Pack your burritos with peppers, onions, and lettuce.

- Add spinach to your soups and pasta sauces.

- Toss peppers, onions, and spinach into your omelets.

Vegetables should fill more than one-third of your plate.

Ordering Chinese? Instead of ordering Chinese chicken and rice, order Chinese broccoli, snow peas, or string beans, with chicken and rice. Fill your stomach with the veggies and eat a little less rice and chicken to save calories.

ways" carbohydrate a "sometimes" or "rarely" one. So stick to the fresh and frozen fruits and vegetables as much as possible.

TIP

DON'T FLIP OVER VEGGIE CHIPS. We all would like to think that anytime a vegetable is mentioned in a food, it is a healthy food. However, this is not always the case. Ounce for ounce, they are very close in calories to their full-fat counterparts. An ounce of regular chips has 150 calories, while Veggie Booty with Spinach and Kale has 130 calories, Good Health Veggie Stix have 140 calories, and an ounce of Terra Stix have 150.

Fresh and frozen fruits and vegetables are actually equally nutritious. If you always come home to wilted vegetables and therefore cannot add them to your meals, you can now turn to frozen ones to top your pizza, toss in your pasta sauce, or throw in your stir-fry, omelet, casserole, or soup.

"Always" carbohydrates contain phytochemicals, which are health-protective nutrients found only in plant foods. Plants naturally produce phytochemicals that protect the plant against disease, and when eaten are believed to enhance the body's natural line of defenses and may help slow the aging process and reduce the risk of cancer, heart disease, stroke, high blood pressure, cataracts, osteoporosis, and urinary tract infections.

Beware: Although you eventually want to aim for ten ½-cup servings of vegetables a day (or more), you don't want to suddenly increase the amount of vegetables you eat, or you may be vulnerable to flatulence, abdominal pain, and diarrhea. So gradually add vegetables into your diet. Start by adding 1 cup more than you are typically eating, then each week add another cup.

And a Cherry on Top

Some people believe that fruits inhibit weight loss because they equate the sweet taste with the harmful effects of concentrated sweets like candy and soda.

Wrong.

When you eat fruits and vegetables, the sugars arrive in the body packaged with fiber, large quantities of water, and many critical vitamins and minerals. On the other hand, all refined sugars, such as those found in candy, enter your body in a concentrated form, spiking your blood sugar and providing few nutrients, if any.

Depending on how many grain servings you are allotted from the table on pages 65 and 66, you should have a specific number of fruit servings. See the list below to discover what is one serving of fruit and how many servings of fruit you need daily in order to fire up your metabolism

One serving from the fruit group is equal to:

- whole fruit such as 1 medium apple, banana, or orange

- ½ grapefruit

- melon wedge (⅛ of melon)

- ½ cup berries

- ½ cup chopped, cooked, or canned fruit

- ¼ cup dried fruit

See list of "always" carbohydrates on pages 23 to 26 for specific fruits.

Notice that fruit juice is not included in the fruit servings—we don't encourage drinking juice. There is no fiber in fruit juice, so it doesn't have the metabolic-revving benefits of real fruit.

TIPS

BLUEBERRIES . . . WHAT A BLESSING! Packed with fiber and antioxidants, blueberries have several bonuses. Animal studies have shown that eating blueberries protects the body from aging, especially in the brain. Blueberries may help prevent urinary tract infections, just as cranberries do.

RACE FOR RAISINS! BUT ONLY ¼ CUP. Calorie-dense raisins are packed with metabolism-revving carbohydrates and plenty of vitamins and minerals. A bonus: Raisins contain powerful antioxidants. Mix them in salads, yogurt, or oatmeal. Or use them to spice up rice and pasta.

WANT A SWEET SNACK? GO FOR BERRIES. A cup of raspberries has eight grams of fiber (four times more than a slice of whole wheat bread). Blackberries are a close second, with seven grams per cup. The fiber slows digestion and keeps the metabolic boost of the carbohydrates in the berries lasting even longer. Mixing berries with "thumbs-up" proteins and the "friendly" fats is the ideal way to fire up your metabolism. Berries can help you to satisfy a sweet tooth craving without adding a lot of calories.

BAN BANANAS? THERE'S ONLY ONE TIME YOU NEED TO DO THIS. Banana chips are fried in artery-clogging oil, and the majority of their calories come from fat, not from metabolism-revving carbohydrates. Fresh bananas, on the other hand, are a nutrient-packed, metabolism-revving sensation.

PINK AND RED ARE BETTER THAN WHITE. GRAPEFRUIT, THAT IS. All fruits and vegetables are great for your health and helping to fire up your metabolism. However, the more color a fruit or veggie has, the more phytochemicals it has. We like to say, "Eat the rainbow of colors," to get the most nutrients.

Daily Fruit Servings

YOUR NUMBER FROM STEP 1 (See page 63)	YOUR LEVEL (To be applied in later chapters)	YOUR DAILY FRUIT SERVINGS
1,200	12	2
1,300	13	2
1,400	14	2
1,500	15	2$\frac{1}{2}$
1,600	16	2$\frac{1}{2}$
1,700	17	2$\frac{1}{2}$
1,800	18	3
1,900	19	3
2,000	20	3
2,100	21	3
2,200	22	3$\frac{1}{2}$
2,300	23	4
2,400	24	4
2,500	25	4
2,600	26	4$\frac{1}{2}$
2,700	27	4$\frac{1}{2}$
2,800	28	5

(continued on next page)

Daily Fruit Servings (cont.)

YOUR NUMBER FROM STEP 1 (See page 63)	YOUR LEVEL (To be applied in later chapters)	YOUR DAILY FRUIT SERVINGS
2,900	29	5
3,000–3,199	30	5½
3,200	31	6
3,300–3,499	32	6
3,500	33	6½

In most cases, you will eat a serving of fruit with a protein serving such as yogurt or with a fat serving like nuts in order to help stave off hunger. However, as an after-dinner snack, you may eat fruit alone.

Energy Bars

Over the past decade, "energy" or power bars have received a lot of hype. Many new clients tell us that they sometimes have two or three bars a day and often use them as meal replacements—after all, they are convenient. And people like eating the bars because they taste like candy bars.

Well, of course they do. Many "energy" bars are the nutritional equivalent of a Snickers. We consider them to be candy-coated vitamin supplements. Since most snack foods are highly processed, contain a lot of added sugars and oils (usually hydrogenated), and contain virtually no fiber, they belong on the "rarely" carbohydrate list and only occasionally on the "sometimes" list. However, if you were going to grab two bags of M&M's from a vending machine for lunch, choosing an energy bar would probably be a better choice, as many bars are fairly low in saturated fat and can have a few grams of fiber and added vitamins and minerals.

HOLD THE BREAD, PLEASE. That's what you need to say whenever you go to a restaurant. Do you usually serve bread before meals when you are eating at home? We hope not, as many people make the mistake of eating more calories from bread before the meal than they should eat for their entire meal. Additionally, most people also eat the grain that is served with the meal, getting more servings of grain at that one sitting than they need for the entire day. Making matters still less metabolically appealing, the bread that is served is almost always a refined grain. This means there is no fiber to fill you up and, therefore, you are even more likely to overeat. So it is best not even to be tempted by bread sitting in front of you; ask that it be left in the kitchen.

EATING CEREAL? DRINK THAT LEFTOVER SKIM OR 1 PERCENT MILK. A significant amount of vitamins (many of which are necessary for a speedy metabolism, as they turn your food into usable energy) from the fortified cereal ends up in the milk.

RICE CAKES A DREAM COME TRUE FOR DIETERS? NOT SO FAST. Although not a bad option, they are usually not whole grain, and some flavors have added sugar. In addition, after munching on rice cakes you may still be craving what you probably were originally looking for—bread. So check your health food stores for whole-grain rice cakes made with brown rice. Or try Hain's Plain Mini Munchies.

Kim's Metabolic Success

Kim came to us in hopes of losing "those last ten pounds." Like that of many clients, her diet contained a lot of refined grains, such as muffins and white rice, and more than the occasional candy, soda, and other "rarely" carbohydrates. Kim had been experiencing energy crashes several times throughout the day and was frequently too exhausted to go to the gym for her evening exercise session.

We immediately started Kim on our Fire Up Your Metabolism plan. Kim replaced many of the refined grains and sugary sweets that she was eating with whole grains. She chose oatmeal for breakfast rather than corn flakes, and exchanged Twizzlers for Ry-Krisp crackers when she wanted a snack. Kim immediately reported that she felt much more satiated (the fiber in the whole-grain products helped to fill her stomach). She was thrilled and reported, "I'm no longer hungry every hour!" In fact, she now wasn't even hungry until her next meal. Even better, she didn't have her usual intense craving for another pack of Twizzlers. And she no longer felt nauseated from a sugar high. What's more, she felt much more energetic and wasn't experiencing energy crashes. Just this one change gave Kim more energy for little simple movements like getting up from her desk, and she also now had plenty of energy to exercise at the end of the day.

Kim lost "those last ten pounds" in five weeks. That was four years ago and the weight is still off.

FOUR

Power Proteins Versus Problem Proteins

Myth Busters

MYTH: If you load up on protein you will be lean and muscular and have great muscle tone.

BUSTED: If you eat more protein than your body needs (if you eat more of anything than your body needs), you will gain body fat, not muscle.

MYTH: If you replace the carbohydrates in your diet with protein, you will have a lot of energy and look great.

BUSTED: Carbohydrates provide your body with energy; protein doesn't. If you replace carbs with protein you will be exhausted, and when you look and feel tired, you don't look good.

MYTH: Most people, and especially vegetarians, don't get enough protein in their diets.

BUSTED: Most people eat far more protein than their bodies require. Even most vegetarians get adequate protein. Many foods other than meat provide good sources of protein.

MYTH: The fat in low-fat and nonfat dairy foods is replaced with chemicals.

BUSTED: Most low-fat and nonfat dairy products use the same ingredients as the full-fat versions, only whole milk is replaced with 1 percent or skim milk.

Our Twin Trial

in which you will witness the benefits of combining proteins and carbs

For this twin trial, we decided that the loser of the coin flip would have to eat a high-protein diet, with limited amounts of carbohydrate, just as many innocent, ill-fated dieters do. We wanted to see just how eating this way would affect us—and our metabolism.

We made sure we didn't change the amount of calories we normally ate, as this would jeopardize our trial—the change in calories, rather than the avoidance of carbohydrates, could influence the results. Instead, we just made sure to eat the amount of protein that "low-carb" diets have you eat, and to limit the carbohydrates that we ate to meet those recommendations as well.

Having witnessed countless clients come to us in desperation after trying very low-carbohydrate diets, we were prepared for the worst. These dieters had warned us: They had lost weight and gained it all back. They had gained back even more weight in some cases. Discouragement, deprivation, and an all-around crummy feeling were common refrains.

So we braced ourselves and held our breath as the coin sailed in the air.

Lyssie: I lost this coin flip. I would be forced to trade my morning breakfast of cereal, soy milk, and fruit for an equal-calorie portion of protein: an egg white omelet with nonfat cheese.

On the first morning of the experiment, I was surprised by how much I enjoyed my omelet. In fact I felt quite satisfied. That is, until midway through my morning exercise bike ride when I suddenly felt exhausted and hot. About forty-five minutes into my normally hour-long bike ride I actually began to feel so weak that I thought I was sick. I went home instead of finishing my workout.

At home I still felt faint and knew that I needed some carbohydrates to replace the muscle energy stores I had just depleted. I plopped down on the couch with a tuna sandwich with mustard. Just as I was about to take a bite, I remembered that during this experiment, I was allowed only a small amount of carbohydrate daily, equivalent to the two slices of bread on the sandwich. (This is actually almost twice the amount of carbohydrates that the Atkins diet allows during its initial phase.) If I ate this sandwich, I couldn't have any more carbohydrates for the rest of the day. I contemplated scraping the tuna from the whole wheat bread and leaving the bread behind, but that was for just a moment—right before I ate the whole thing.

After all, I was sick!

Several minutes later, I was feeling much better, and within about a half hour, I was back to normal. In fact, I got angry with myself for not finishing my workout and thinking I had been sick. I should have known that my dizziness and exhaustion were due to having the wrong kind of fuel for my body—protein. I had felt hot and overheated because I had perceived my workout to be too difficult when in fact I was just inadequately fueled. I decided to return to the gym later in the day.

I spent the rest of the day contemplating the challenge of figuring out what to eat. My next meal consisted of a chicken breast on a bed of lettuce with ½ cup of cottage cheese and low-fat string cheese. As midafternoon rolled around, I realized that I wasn't hungry for a midafternoon snack. Although this was nice, on the flip side, I was also tired and sluggish, and later in the day quite shaky. That night for dinner I had grilled fish and some vegetables. (This continued to be my usual dinner during the course of this experiment—fish, turkey, or chicken with veggies.)

The next morning I woke up feeling as though I hadn't even slept. I decided that I would need to eat my carbohydrate portion in the morning so that I could get through my exercise routine. My workout was easier than it had seemed the day before; however, it still felt much more challenging than usual, and I could not pedal as quickly. As the day continued and I was primarily fueling myself with protein, the sluggishness set in again. The only thing I could think about was sleep. I nodded off six times during the day! I had a hard time getting up from my desk to make photocopies. I was craving sleep.

There was also something else I was craving—carbohydrates. My carbohydrate cravings couldn't have been worse. You can't imagine how much restraint I had to use at lunch when I ate my tuna and turkey "sandwiches" on lettuce instead of on bread. Several days I actually had to drag my exhausted body out of my house just so that I wouldn't ruin the trial by diving into a loaf of bread. And things worsened as the day crept on. What fun were my snacks—cheese without crackers? By the time dinners rolled around, I would nearly cry staring at the hunk of fish, chicken, or turkey on my otherwise seemingly empty plate. What I would have done for pasta, rice, bread, or a potato. I was ready to sell my left kidney for just a couple of bites of bread or a Snyder's hard pretzel.

And one other thing. I wish I didn't have to mention it, but it's an issue for anyone who eats a high-protein, very low-carb diet: constipation. I finally know what this word means, literally, since I experienced it, despite eating decent portions of vegetables. "What do you mean I can't have prune juice?" I would have never dreamed that these words would come out of my mouth, but thanks to the carb restrictions, they did, as prune juice contains too many carbs for this trial. I now understand why my grandma drinks it. I would drink or eat anything to prevent the discomfort of constipation, too.

The only good thing about this experiment was that I never really felt too hungry. However, I never felt healthy or energetic either, and especially not during my exercise, which I still dragged myself to do anyway, only at a much slower pace than usual. I convinced Tammy to allow this experiment to last only three weeks.

I was relieved to be done with the experiment—and crestfallen to learn that in just twenty-one days my body fat increased 1 percent even though my calorie intake was the same as it was before the trial.

The reason: I felt so lifeless during the whole trial that I didn't burn off nearly as many calories through exercise and everyday activity as I usually burn when my body gets the fuel it needs.

Unfortunately, I didn't gain muscle either. Instead, since I had not fed my body the carbohydrates it needed for energy, my body was forced to use some protein I was eating to get energy, stealing it from its real job—assisting in muscle growth. In fact, since my weight remained the same yet my body fat increased, that signified that I had actually *lost* muscle (my fatigue prevented me from completing my normal strength-training routine) and worse still, I had gained body fat and slowed my metabolic rate. My muscles looked less shapely, particularly in my arms.

On the bright side, I have to say that the next morning, my granola, soy milk, and fruit had never tasted so good, and my workout had never seemed easier and more fun!

Protein Propaganda

Protein bars, protein shakes, protein powders, protein drinks. Protein seems to be all the rage. Shelves nationwide are stocked with the latest popular protein supplements. Fueled by all of this hype, everyone from stay-at-home moms and weekend exercisers to professional athletes comes into our office for the first time with many misconceptions about what these protein supplements will and will not do for them. Some clients tell us that they eat an afternoon protein bar to give them energy and to keep them lean. We repeatedly hear many of the same comments and questions:

"I don't love the way this protein bar tastes, but I should eat it because it's good for me, right?"

"I heard this protein drink will make me lean. It will, won't it?"

"If I take this protein powder three times a day like the container says, it will help me to build muscle, right?"

Everyone wants to hear the same thing: Eating a protein bar or drinking a shake will make them stronger and leaner and able to perform better.

Well, here's the truth: Don't waste your time and money on these protein supplements. They will not make you stronger or firmer. Nor do they provide any benefit over eating a protein-containing food. In fact, foods that contain protein provide many benefits over the protein supplement, such as giving you the vitamins and minerals that naturally occur in the food, as well as making you feel full. Not to mention, it is easy to get all of the protein you need from real food, and it is a lot more flavorful and a lot less expensive. So instead of protein supplements, you should choose the right protein-rich foods at the right time; this will fire up your metabolism and help you to look the way you want to. In order to understand why certain proteins must be chosen at certain times, you must first know a little bit about protein and the way it works in your body.

What Does Protein Do for Me?

Protein is the main component of muscles, organs, and glands. Every living cell and all body fluids, except bile and urine, contain protein. Protein helps blood to clot by plugging cuts and scrapes with fibrin, a stringy mass of protein fibers. If it weren't for protein, a pinprick could drain your body of all your blood. Protein maintains the cells of muscles, tendons, and ligaments and helps to control your body's fluid balance by regulating the quantity of fluids inside the blood vessels, inside the cells, and surrounding the cells. It also helps maintain the body's acid-base balance, which is critical—if the blood gets either too acidic or too basic, life cannot be sustained as protein becomes denatured and cannot carry out any of its functions, causing bodily processes to fail.

Why Is Protein Essential for a Speedy Metabolism?

Remember, your metabolic rate is the speed at which your body burns calories.

Protein helps build and repair muscle broken down from activity and exercise. This is *huge*—the more muscle you have, the more calories your body burns. The presence of muscle alone burns calories because it is metabolically active; this means muscle uses calories even while your body is at rest.

Protein also revs your metabolism by slowing down the digestion of carbohydrates. Protein is digested more slowly than carbohydrates, so when you mix carbohydrates with a little bit of protein, the protein causes the carbohydrates to digest more gradually, giving you an even energy flow. As you may remember from Chapters 2 and 3, carbohydrates provide the body with glucose, the primary fuel for the brain and muscles. The presence of carbohydrates prevents the body from feeling threatened and using your "calorie-burning" muscle tissue for fuel. However, as you also learned in Chapter 3, when carbohydrates are eaten alone (especially the "sometimes" or "rarely" ones), glucose (fuel) quickly enters your bloodstream, causing your pancreas to kick out an abnormally large amount of insulin, the hormone whose job it is to quickly shuttle the glucose out of the blood and into the tissues and muscles. This large surge of insulin results in your blood sugar level dropping quickly. As your blood sugar level dips, so does your energy level. Immediately, your brain realizes that your blood sugar is low and it sends the signal to your body to get more fuel . . . and so you eat.

Therefore, in the absence of a small amount of protein, carbohydrates *cannot* fire up the metabolism to its ultimate potential; the

You *can* prevent sugar highs and crashes, and the subsequent overeating that results from white carbs and/or sugar, by eating a serving of protein with that carbohydrate. For example, eat that serving of white rice with 2 ounces of chicken breast mixed in it. Eat that slice of bread with a slice (³/₄ ounce) of low-fat cheese on top. This carbohydrate and protein combination will wake you up in the afternoon and provide more sustained energy than that candy bar. Having some protein will help you to feel satisfied for an extended period of time, and what's more, your body will continue to burn calories, as well, by providing you with longer-lasting energy.

calorie-burning blast is short-lived. What's more, without a little bit of protein, the surge of insulin released may trigger you to overeat.

What Happens If I Don't Eat Protein at My Meals?

Some clients come to us wondering why they always seem to be hungry shortly after finishing their meals. Actually, "ravenous" is the word they use. They claim that this hunger causes them to snack excessively and to consume extra calories. Debbie, for example, wanted to lose her "last six pounds" and return to her prepregnancy weight. Debbie's diet consisted of fruit and whole wheat toast with jam for breakfast; a large salad of greens with croutons, mixed vegetables, and nonfat dressing at lunch; and a small plate of pasta for dinner. Every hour or two, Debbie would get hungry, so she would snack on fruit, pretzels, frozen yogurt, and/or an occasional piece of candy. Although this is a seemingly healthy diet, and very similar to that of many Americans who are diligently trying to watch their weight, it is missing a key ingredient when it comes to speeding up your metabolic rate.

Protein.

None of Debbie's foods provided her with a significant amount of it. Without protein, the carbs Debbie was eating could not satisfy her nearly as long as they could had they been mixed with a bit of protein. Within one day of replacing the jam on her toast with some lowfat cottage cheese, exchanging the croutons on her lunchtime salad for tofu slices, and adding chicken to a smaller plate of pasta at dinner, Debbie no longer needed more than two or three snacks a day. Within three weeks, she had lost those six pounds and she has kept them off ever since.

TIPS

AN APPETIZER OF MISO SOUP? THAT'S A BALL THAT GOES RIGHT THROUGH THE HOOP. Most appetizers are loaded with fat and calories. Although miso soup is quite high in sodium, it is low in calories and provides you with a little bit of a great source of protein, tofu.

EATING ITALIAN? The Chicken Marsala is one of your best bets. It uses the lean chicken breast, and a typical ten-ounce portion has 460 calories and only seven grams of "bad" fat—not bad for a restaurant meal. Keep in mind that ten ounces may be all the protein you need for the entire day, so don't eat it all in one sitting. If you get this much, take home half for tomorrow.

I Lift Weights, So Where Are My Muscles?

Like Debbie, a handful of clients come to us as protein conservatives, yet they have a different issue from hunger pangs. These clients exercise and lift weights but never seem to see the muscle tone or definition they are looking for. After making sure that these clients include a few more protein sources in their diet, these former "protein neglecters" are thrilled by their results as they finally see the body they work so hard for.

After reading this, many of you are probably going to add protein liberally to your plate. *Not so fast.* Being too extreme one way or another can ultimately fizzle rather than fire up your metabolism.

TIPS

BUYING GROUND BEEF? IT HAD BETTER BE A DARK, DEEP RED— WITHOUT EVEN A HINT OF PINK! If your ground beef is pink, there is a lot of white (fat) mixed in with the red (lean meat [protein]).

BAN BACON, UNLESS IT'S CANADIAN OR TURKEY BACON. Just 2½ ounces of bacon (half the size of your palm) has 410 calories and thirty-five grams of fat (twelve of them are saturated), which is close to the maximum amount of artery-clogging saturated fat that you should get in an entire day. Regular bacon is about the worst thing you can eat. However, you can eat Canadian bacon or turkey bacon, which are lean, "thumbs-up" proteins. If you choose extralean turkey bacon or extra-lean Canadian bacon, you could have three slices for around the same calories as two slices of the regular turkey bacon or Canadian bacon. If you must eat bacon (a "thumbs-down" protein), eat just one slice.

DON'T EVEN THINK ABOUT GROUND TURKEY . . . UNLESS IT'S THE BREAST. Many people assume that ground turkey is leaner than ground beef because it's turkey, a supposedly healthy meat. Unfortunately, their good intentions backfire and they often get more calories and fat than if they had eaten red meat. That's because if it doesn't say ground turkey *breast,* you can bet that the skin and fattier parts of the bird are ground in there—tripling the fat and calories. Be sure to buy the ground *breast* of the turkey and avoid plain ground turkey.

PORTION DISTORTION. Never sit down to more than a palm-size (about five to six ounces) portion of protein, which is the maximum amount of meat that inactive people need each day. The United States Department of Agriculture (USDA) recommends a maximum of six to nine ounces of meat a day, depending on your total calorie requirements. It is easy to go to a restaurant and get eight to nine ounces at just one meal! So put your hand next to your meat portion so you can see how it compares to the size of your palm (fingers not included). If it is bigger than your palm, cut away the excess and put it on your bread plate. Immediately ask your server to put it in a doggy bag or just take it away. That way it won't tempt you.

BRAIN TEASER: When does 80 percent lean = 70 percent fat? When it comes to ground beef. Don't be tricked by "lean" or "extra-lean" ground beef labeled with its fat content, such as "10 percent fat" or, on the other hand, "90 percent lean." This is the percentage of fat by weight, not the "percentage of calories" from fat. Expressing fat by weight is misleading. If the meat is labeled 80 percent lean, 20 percent of its total weight is fat, which is equal to 70 percent of the total calories coming from fat. Meat that is labeled "10 percent fat" actually has 51 percent of its calories from fat. If it says "25 percent fat," then 75 percent of its calories come from fat!

As you now understand, leaving either carbohydrates or protein out of your diet is detrimental to firing up your metabolism. And eating too much of one nutrient crowds out the other, also causing problems. However, by following our Fire Up Your Metabolism plan, your success in revving up your metabolic engine is guaranteed when you stick to your specific number of servings and the appropriate serving size; you can be certain that you are not overeating any one nutrient. Remember, eating more of anything than your body needs, even protein, results in a gain in body fat, not a gain in lean muscle tissue.

What Happens When I Get Too Much Protein in My Diet?

We hate to have to be the protein police, but there are several things you should know before you have an omelet for breakfast, a chicken sandwich for lunch, and a steak for dinner.

First, when you consume more protein than you need, as the average American does, you crowd out your metabolism-revving carbohydrates, so your body starts the arduous, metabolism-inefficient task of using protein for fuel.

But more than anything, a diet that is too high in protein makes you tired. Protein takes a long time to digest (about four to six hours versus one half to four hours to digest and burn up carbohydrates). Although protein's slower digestion rate can be a good thing (it promotes satiety when you combine the right amounts of the best carbohydrates with the appropriate portions of the best proteins), it can also be a negative thing when you overdo it because a large portion of blood leaves the brain and muscles and stays in your stomach (and intestine) for a long period of time for digestion. This means that there is less blood available to supply the muscles and brain with oxygen, causing sluggishness and decreased energy. In addition, too much protein in the diet can lead to high cholesterol (many foods that are high

Need help counting your servings? Here's an example. After following our steps you see that you need six carbohydrate servings a day. You decide to have a cheese sandwich for lunch. This has two slices of bread, which is equal to two carbohydrate servings. You know that when you eat a grain serving, you need to eat a protein (or fat) serving too. So in this case it would be ideal to eat two protein servings. One protein serving from part-skim mozzarella cheese is the size of one pointer finger, so you can have two pointer-finger-size servings of cheese on your sandwich. Then, after eating this cheese sandwich, you will have had two grain servings and two protein servings.

in protein are also high in the artery–clogging saturated fat and/or cholesterol) or calcium loss from the bone, promoting osteoporosis or other diseases, such as gout. High–protein diets may also put a strain on your kidneys and liver, as these two organs are responsible for breaking down protein and then excreting the excess nitrogen that is created from the protein.

The trick to firing up your metabolism is balancing your intake of proteins and carbs.

TIPS

SURPRISE! A RED MEAT THAT'S LEANER THAN CHICKEN. Buffalo is actually a red meat that's leaner than most. Three ounces of buffalo have just 111 calories and 1.5 grams of fat. Even the leanest parts of the cow, such as the loin and the round, have about 180 calories and 7.5 grams of fat in the same-size serving. So if you enjoy the flavor of red meat, try buffalo.

ROTISSERIE CHICKEN ISN'T AS GOOD FOR YOU AS YOU MAY THINK. Usually, when you cook chicken, the fat drips off, but rotisserie chicken keeps turning and the fat drips right back into the chicken.

GOOD-BYE, CHICKEN POT PIE. This meal usually uses the fatty dark meat. Making matters worse, the pastry dough is loaded with butter. Things don't get any better when it comes to the sauce, which is usually made of cream.

EATING CHINESE? ALWAYS SPECIFY THAT YOU WANT WHITE MEAT CHICKEN. Otherwise you're sure to get the very fatty, dark meat, which can almost double the calories in your meal.

How Can I Get the Right Amount of Protein?

Follow our guidelines to get the right mix of protein and carbohydrates so that you will be like our clients who have fired up their metabolism.

Your daily grain servings (as determined in Chapter 3) equal your daily protein servings. Also refer to the "thumbs-up" and "thumbs-down" protein lists on pages 33 to 37 to see which list your favorite proteins are on and what constitutes a serving.

You can be sure that you're getting just the right amount of protein to fire up your metabolism by matching the number of your daily grain servings to your daily protein servings. For example, if you are allowed six grain servings daily, you are allowed six protein servings. (This should make it easier for you to remember how many servings you need.) Just be careful how you count them: Add up only your grain carbohydrates, not vegetables and fruits, when you are matching your protein servings. Remember, you can eat vegetables in unlimited quantities (just be sure to get a minimum of 4½ servings). And you can find how many servings of fruit you need on pages 73 to 74.

Simply remember how many carbohydrate servings you are allotted; your ability to rev up your metabolism is ultimately centered on your total carbohydrate servings. So just by keeping track of the number of grains your body requires for a speedy metabolism, you ensure that you are getting the right amount of protein, and you will fire up your metabolism.

Daily Protein Servings

YOUR NUMBER FROM STEP 1 (See page 63)	YOUR LEVEL (To be applied in later chapters)	YOUR DAILY PROTEIN SERVINGS
1,200	12	5
1,300	13	5
1,400	14	5
1,500	15	5
1,600	16	6
1,700	17	6
1,800	18	6
1,900	19	7
2,000	20	$7^1/_2$
2,100	21	8
2,200	22	8
2,300	23	8
2,400	24	9
2,500	25	10
2,600	26	10
2,700	27	11
2,800	28	11
2,900	29	$11^1/_2$
3,000–3,199	30	$11^1/_2$
3,200	31	$11^1/_2$
3,300–3,499	32	12
3,500	33	12

It will take about a week for you to get accustomed to the serving sizes and to matching your protein servings and grain servings. Don't worry so much about getting an equal number of protein and grain servings at the same sitting. Instead, just be sure that you do not eat a grain without some protein or vice versa (or some fat), and that at the end of the day you have gotten the appropriate servings of each. Keep your food diary so that you can be sure that you have met your requirements at the end of the day. Soon this will become second nature.

To ensure that you boost your metabolism to your utmost ability, you will never eat a grain by itself, even for a snack. Instead, you will couple it with a protein that you have chosen from the protein list on pages 33 to 35 (or with a fat, which we discuss in the next chapter). It is okay to eat a vegetable or a fruit by itself for a snack. Just make sure that you will be eating a larger meal within one to two hours, as the fruit or vegetable will neither satiate you nor provide you with energy for very long.

When you choose a protein, you will then use the Rule of Hand (see page 92) to apply the correct protein portion size to the carbohydrate serving you eat. Ideally, if you eat two servings of carbohydrates at one sitting, you also should aim to eat two servings of protein from the protein list. However, this is not always possible, so just remember to stick to your total daily servings of each grain and protein.

Remember, you do not need to eat only one serving at one sitting—just be sure to count how many servings you eat over the course of the day. If some people sat down to a meal with one protein serving, not only would they be hungry, but they would never get all of their servings in over the course of the day.

The Rule of Hand

The foods that contain protein are divided into two categories: powerful proteins, which receive the "thumbs-up"; and perilous proteins, which receive the "thumbs-down."

To get started, combine your carbohydrate choice with any of the options from the "Thumbs-Up" Powerful Proteins list on pages 33 to 35 in Chapter 2, and stick to the Rule of Hand. Each protein is listed with its part of the hand-size portion. The "thumbs-up" proteins have been carefully selected, as they are the best protein options for combining with carbohydrates. The "thumbs-up" options are ideal for firing up your metabolism because they are lean protein sources (low in fat) and, therefore, in their appropriate portion sizes they will adequately extend the metabolism-revving boost of the carbohydrates. What's more, since these protein portions are moderate size, and because they are low in fat, they don't overwhelm your system by causing the blood to stay in the stomach for too long, competing with your blood supply to your muscles. Therefore, you will have plenty of energy to be active and burn calories. And although it takes a little bit of practice to get accustomed to the serving sizes of each, soon, after using the Rule of Hand, it becomes easy.

TIPS

TIRED OF CHICKEN? TAKE A WALK ON THE WILD SIDE. Try ostrich, which, like chicken, is poultry. This bird has gained a lot of popularity as a healthy alternative to the same old chicken. Chicken breast has about 140 calories and three grams of fat in a three-ounce serving. Ostrich has 108 calories and two to three grams of fat in the same-size serving. (Three ounces is about the size of a deck of cards or the size of four fingers.)

A "THUMBS-DOWN" PROTEIN CAN BECOME A "THUMBS-UP" ONE. Here's how to remove about half the fat from ground beef.

1) Start with the reddest, leanest meat possible. 2) Brown it in a skillet. 3) Place cooked meat on paper towels. 4) Dump meat into a strainer and rinse it with hot (not boiling) water. 5) Drain it completely.

Choosing the Best Proteins

Many protein foods, such as many of the "thumbs-down" proteins, contain saturated fat, which raises your cholesterol level and is responsible for making your blood "sticky." "Sticky" cells are more likely to clump together and clot, or become part of the plaque in artery walls, thereby contributing to heart disease. (What's more, although it has not yet been scientifically tested, we believe that anything that hampers smooth flow of blood and oxygen throughout your body and to your working muscles also negatively impacts your body processes, including your metabolic rate.) The "thumbs-up" proteins such as white meat chicken and turkey without the skin are much lower in artery-clogging saturated fat and are much healthier than beef, lamb, or most cuts of pork. Protein foods like fish, soy products, nonfat and low-fat dairy products, and especially beans have many health benefits.

Fish

By far, the best meat to eat is fish. Fish have omega-3 fatty acids that protect the heart by reducing the clotting tendency of the blood and reducing the risk of heart attack and stroke. The omega-3s in fish may also help to maintain a normal heart rhythm and may lower triglycerides. As strange as it may seem, the fish that have the most of these benefits are the ones that are highest in fat (the omega-3 fatty acids), such as salmon, herring, anchovies, oysters, sardines, whitefish, and mackerel.

TIPS

SEARCH FOR SCALLOPS. Scallops are low in fat and high in protein, and they are sure to fire up your metabolism when served on a small bed of brown rice with vegetables.

FRIED FISH? FISH FOR SOMETHING ELSE. Eating fish with an "always" carbohydrate is one of the best ways to extend the metabolic boost from that carbohydrate food. However, if your fish swam in oil on its way to your plate, kiss it good-bye. Eating fried fish overwhelms your metabolism, leaving you a lethargic, calorie-hoarding rather than calorie-burning machine. Eat your fish baked, steamed, grilled, poached, or even cooked in wine, just steer clear of it fried, and you'll be just fine.

TRY THE TUNA! Grilled, poached, steamed, topped with teriyaki sauce, or wrapped in seaweed in your favorite sushi roll, tuna is sure to please. Note: To fire up your metabolism, when you buy canned tuna, be sure that it is canned in water and not in oil.

GIVE TUNA SALAD A TUNE-UP. To save your waistline, instead of using regular, calorie-dense, fat-packed mayonnaise, use mustard or nonfat or low-fat mayonnaise as your dressing.

GETTING BORED? TRY THE SWORD! Swordfish has only 150 calories per three-ounce serving and a healthy dose of omega-3s. Try preparing this fish with a summer salsa made with chopped tomatoes, cucumbers, apples, and bell peppers.

SUSHI IS SUPER—UNLESS IT IS THE SPICY ROLLS, THEN STEER CLEAR! The fish in sushi gives you your "thumbs-up" protein. Unfortunately, the spicy rolls have a mayonnaise sauce, which makes this healthy protein an artery-clogging, fatty meal.

Mercury in Fish

Recently, the Food and Drug Administration warned women in their childbearing years to avoid certain fish, including swordfish, shark, king mackerel, and tilefish, as they contain concentrated levels of mercury. The FDA is being urged to target tuna, both raw and canned, as also being high in mercury and potentially harmful to a fetus's devel-

Include fish in your diet at least two times per week. You will benefit from their omega-3 fats, which help to lower cholesterol and
help prevent your blood from becoming too "sticky."

oping nervous system. So if you are a woman of childbearing age,
stick to the fish/seafood with the lowest levels of mercury: blue crab,
farmed-raised catfish, croaker (not white), flounder, haddock, salmon
(both farm-raised and wild), shrimp, and farm-raised trout.

TIPS

LOBSTER, PREPARED IN WHITE WINE, IS JUST FINE. Lobster is a
"thumbs-up" protein that is usually made a "thumbs-down" protein
by being dunked in butter. Butter adds one hundred calories per
level tablespoon. So cook it in white wine and the lobster won't add
an ounce to your behind. And say yes to lobster if it's dipped in
lemon and cocktail sauce.

SHRIMP TEMPURA? WHAT A HORROR! After the shrimp are bat-
tered and fried, they have more than twice the calories as grilled
shrimp.

EATING THAI? TRY THE SHRIMP SHUMAI. Steamed and not fried,
this dish is packed with shrimp's "thumbs-up" protein.

STEAMED CRAB? HOW FAB! This "thumbs-up" protein is low in fat
and calories. Go to a Maryland crab feast, and with a little wishful
thinking you may even burn more calories than you eat by cracking
open the crab shells.

CRAB CAKE? BIG MISTAKE. Not only are crab cakes usually prepared with tons of mayo, they are then deep-fried. Save your
waistline and go for the lump or fresh crabmeat, which are
"thumbs-up" metabolism-revving proteins.

BE A FAN OF STEAMED MUSSELS AND STEAMED CLAMS. Both are "thumbs-up" proteins that are sure to give your metabolism a boost when combined with an "always" carbohydrate.

FILLET OF SOLE IS GOOD FOR YOUR SOUL. You'll feel good after eating this fish, knowing that you just ate a "thumbs-up" protein-packed, low-fat fish. As with all foods, just be sure it isn't fried. And be sure to have a metabolism-revving "always" carbohydrate, such as a small baked potato, with it.

Soy

Soy and its products are some of the best protein options. As dietitians, we have heard people say that just the thought of including soy foods into their meal plans makes them cringe, although usually they admit to having never even tried any soy foods. When we tell them that they probably have already unknowingly welcomed it onto their plates—in miso soup, in smoothies or fruit shakes, in omelets, in Chinese dishes, or in the edamame (green pea pods) that are served at Japanese restaurants—they realize that their fear is unfounded.

- Add soy milk to your soups and cereals and vanilla soy milk to hot chocolate.

- Sprinkle soy nuts on your salad or in your yogurt.

- Try soy sausage links, soy burgers, or soy cheese.

- Spread soy butter (similar to peanut butter) on your sandwich.

- Puree tofu and blend it with your favorite dip mix such as onion or ranch, or mix it with ricotta in your favorite lasagna recipe.

- Did someone mention pie? You can make a cheesecake pie by using pureed silken tofu as a substitute for some of the cream cheese.

Soy protein can lower your body's "bad" LDL cholesterol. What's more, it may keep your blood vessels healthy because one of the components in soy, called genistein, helps to prevent blood from clumping and clotting (clumping narrows the vessels and leads to clogged arteries and heart disease). A bonus: Including soy in your diet may reduce the risk of other chronic diseases like cancer and osteoporosis. The great news is that you don't have to give up eating beef or chicken to reap the benefits of this "thumbs-up" protein. Just make a few adjustments in some of your favorite meals to include soy products. For example, in a sloppy joe, use half ground beef and half soy crumbles.

TIPS

MAKE IT CRUMBLE. Soy meat crumbles are easy to include in your meals to make a lower-calorie, heart-healthy dish. Cook sloppy joes, lasagna, and spaghetti and meat sauce with this tasty alternative to high-fat meat. Find soy crumbles in the frozen section of your grocery store. And while you're there, be sure to pick up a soy burger. Try Boca Burgers, which are a favorite of our clients. One original burger is one protein serving.

BRING ME EDAMAME. This green pea pod often served at Japanese restaurants is a soybean. It is one of our clients' favorite appetizers. It is surely one of the healthiest appetizers and one of the few ways that you can actually get fiber when you eat protein! Each $^2/_3$-cup serving, with shells, is one "thumbs-up" protein.

HOT DIGGITY DOG! Yes, you can have a hot dog, but only if it is a soy hot dog. And while you're at it, give a nod to soy sausage. Our clients love Morningstar Farms brand.

Believing in the Bean

Beans are loaded with iron, folic acid, and fiber, all of which many Americans are deficient in. Also filled with protein and potassium, lentils, pinto beans, and garbanzos (not green beans or wax beans), have been shown to lower cholesterol within three to four weeks when eaten by people with elevated cholesterol levels.

TIPS

DON'T BEAN SHY. All you need is ¹/₂ cup. In addition to being a great source of protein, beans are a source of "always" carbs. So beans are the entire metabolic-revving package in themselves. They contain carbohydrates to provide you with energy to be active. They also have fiber to help you to feel satiated and to make the metabolic-revving and energy boost of the carbohydrates last longer. (A bowl of beans has more fiber than your basic high-fiber cereal.) What's more, they are packed with protein that will extend the metabolic boost of the carbohydrates. So don't bean shy! Aim for ¹/₂ cup three times a week. Order a bean burrito at a Mexican restaurant (just be sure the beans aren't refried). Try lentil soup or bean chili. Sprinkle beans in your salad, and dip your veggies in hummus or a low-fat bean dip.

REFRIED IS USUALLY A SIN, BUT IT DOESN'T HAVE TO BE. Choose Bearitos or Old El Paso fat-free refried beans. These beans have the texture and taste of their lard-ridden counterparts. Roll up ¹/₂ cup of these beans and some chopped bell peppers in a small whole wheat tortilla and sprinkle with nonfat cheese and salsa. Then microwave, and voilà! You have a healthy lunch, snack, or dinner. Remember, just ¹/₂ cup is all it takes to have a great dose of metabolism protein and fiber! (Note: More is not better.)

LIVE FOR THE LENTIL. But only ¹/₂ cup. A ¹/₂-cup serving contains a whopping eight grams of fiber, nine grams of protein, and virtually no fat. And lentils are like other beans in that they provide a metabolic boost with a satiating burst of nutrients, especially folate and iron.

Dairy

Nonfat and low-fat dairy products round out the "thumbs-up" protein list. The key is choosing *nonfat* and *low-fat* dairy products rather than reduced-fat and whole-milk dairy products, which are high in saturated fat and calories.

A study at Purdue University found a connection between calcium and weight loss in women. Women who consumed the highest levels of calcium lost more body fat than women with calcium-deficient diets.

TIPS

REDUCED-FAT CHEESE IS NOT AS LOW IN FAT AS IT SOUNDS. Reduced-fat just means 25 percent less fat than the original product, so it is still high in fat. Choose low-fat and nonfat cheese. Avoid cheese in meals at restaurants when you can't ensure that you are getting low-fat and nonfat varieties. This little adjustment alone has terrific results.

DID YOU THINK FARMER'S CHEESE WAS LOW-FAT? THINK AGAIN. This fresh cheese is a form of cottage cheese from which most of the liquid has been pressed. It contains one hundred calories per ounce and eight grams of fat (six of which are saturated). For an item to qualify as a "low-fat" food, it must contain fewer than three grams of fat per serving. So this cheese is far from low-fat.

AVOIDING PIZZA? Here's one that won't sabotage your efforts to fire up your metabolism. One slice of Pizza Hut's Hand Tossed Veggie Lover's Pizza has 180 calories and five grams of fat (only two grams of fat are the artery-clogging kind).

Our clients love snacking on low-fat string cheese or nonfat and low-fat yogurt and cottage cheese. Add nonfat cheese varieties to burritos, lasagna, mashed potatoes, soups, and other combination dishes. There is a bonus to eating low-fat and nonfat yogurt: Yogurt has enough carbohydrates and protein to provide your body with the benefits of both carbohydrates and protein; it doesn't have to be mixed with more carbohydrate, protein, or fat in order to fire up your metabolism. Yogurt can be eaten alone for a metabolism-revving snack.

TIPS

HERE'S HOW TO KEEP SKIM MILK SKINNY YET BUFF. You say that skim milk is too watery? Try Skim Plus or add a teaspoon or two of nonfat dried milk to each cup. Skim Plus is the same as skim milk but with added calcium and a consistency more like whole milk. You get a thicker and richer-tasting milk with more calcium and protein yet not more fat.

THINK TWICE ABOUT HALF-AND-HALF. Just ½ cup of half-and-half has 160 calories and thirteen grams of fat, and nine of those fat grams are saturated. Eighty percent of half-and-half's calories come from fat, not from protein. On the other hand, Land O' Lakes fat-free half-and-half, made from skim milk and a little carrageen (added to make a creamy texture), is a "thumbs-up" protein that can fire up your metabolism. And it can revolutionize fettuccine Alfredo.

EAT YOGURT, BE LEAN? NOT SO FAST. Most people assume that yogurt and cottage cheese are the original weight-loss foods. However, some regular fruit-flavored yogurts have a whopping 250 to 280 calories in just one cup (eight ounces). And if it's not skim or 1 percent cottage cheese, it can actually cause you to pack on the pounds. When it comes to yogurt, look for the nonfat light yogurt, which has just 120 calories in a cup, or plain nonfat yogurt, which has 110 calories in a cup. For cottage cheese, have ½ cup of the nonfat or 1 percent fat cottage cheese and you will get one hundred calories.

LOVE CREAMY YOGURT? Fat-free Greek yogurt has a deliciously thick and creamy texture, yet with no fat. Look for it at specialty markets and Greek markets.

Eggs

Accused of raising the body's cholesterol level, the egg has gotten a rotten rep. Recently, however, eggs were given a clean slate, as they contain only 1¹/₂ grams of saturated fat, the main dietary culprit for raising blood cholesterol levels. They are a healthy "thumbs-up" protein and can help you jump-start your metabolism. Combining one whole egg or several egg whites with an "always" carbohydrate is a surefire way to feel satiated while firing up your metabolism by extending the metabolic boost from the carbohydrate. Just remember, moderation is the key. (If you have high cholesterol, limit egg yolks to three per week.)

WAKEY, WAKEY . . . EGGS AND OATMEAL. For the ultimate Fire Up Your Metabolism breakfast, have two scrambled egg whites (cooked in cooking spray, of course!) and one cup of cooked oatmeal.

EGGS IN A BROWN BAG? Absolutely, when you're talkin' hard-boiled. Your midafternoon snack is easy to pack—just toss a hard-boiled egg and ten Health Valley Whole Wheat crackers in a brown bag for a great carbohydrate-protein combination.

THERE ARE A FEW TIMES TO SAY NO TO SALAD. Egg salad, chicken salad, tuna salad, and whitefish salad are all loaded with mayonnaise. Therefore, most of the calories in these salads come from fat and not from the protein found in eggs, chicken, and fish. Steer clear!

Don't Deny Yourself

Chances are you love at least some of the "thumbs-down" foods. Don't deny yourself. Just be cautious with the portion size. Portions of "thumbs-down" proteins should be one-half the size of their "thumbs-up" counterparts. We realize that these portions are probably smaller than you are accustomed to, but the point is that you can eat these foods as long as you limit yourself. Here's what to do: Limit the "thumbs-down" options to seven servings each week. You can have these servings any time you choose. This means that you can have all seven servings in a splurge day, or you can have one serving every day.

How would you count a pizza? Don't let combination foods stump you. Just break them down. For pizza, ask yourself how many pieces of bread the dough equals. (A slice of most large pizzas is equal to about 1½ slices of bread.) Therefore, a slice of pizza is 1½ grain servings. Then determine how much cheese is on the pizza. (We recommend that you ask for "light" on the cheese if you order your pizza from a restaurant, as full-fat cheese is high in calories and fat. Also, blot the oil off the cheese with a napkin to save your waistline and hundreds of calories. Every tablespoon you blot off saves you 120 calories.) Then, use the Rule of Hand to help you to determine how many servings of protein you get from the cheese. Remember, when it comes to full-fat cheese, 1 serving is the size (thickness and length) of your pointer finger. If you didn't order your pizza "light on the cheese," chances are that one slice could give you 3½ to 4 protein servings. If this is the case, you may want to pull off some of the fatty cheese. As for the tomato sauce, if no oil has been added in the preparation, it counts as a veggie. We recommend filling your stomach by ordering extra veggies on the pizza. So if you ordered a veggie pizza, "light on the cheese," you'll eat about 1½ grain servings, 2 protein servings and 2 vegetable servings.

FIVE

Favoring Fabulous Fats

Myth Busters

MYTH: Olive oil is the healthiest oil and should be used liberally.

BUSTED: Although olive oil is a healthy oil and is good for your heart, it shouldn't be used liberally. It is easy to add five hundred calories or more to your meal by cooking your food in olive oil. Each tablespoon contains 120 calories. If it isn't limited, it will cause weight gain.

MYTH: All fats are bad for you.

BUSTED: All fats are not bad for you. In fact, eating some fat is essential for good health. Fat is necessary to absorb fat-soluble vitamins, keep skin soft and looking young, and add satiety to your meals.

Aaaaah . . . the thought of devouring a warm, rich chocolate brownie as it melts in your mouth, or the cool, refreshing feeling of ice cream as it slides down your throat. Or for some, the true luxury is diving into that juicy hamburger. We love fat in our food, yet we despise it on our thighs, hips, and waists.

Clients come to us with varying ideas about how much fat they should allow in their diets. Some are extremists, "fatphobics" who have completely turned their back on all fats, fearing that the fat they eat will make them fat. Some indulge in fatty food after fatty food, believing that it is the carbohydrates that make them fat. While still others are more moderate, indulging in fatty foods because they taste too good to give up, yet trying to limit the portion sizes of these "indulgences" in the hopes of keeping the fat on their body at bay.

You are probably wondering which of these clients has the right approach. Before we answer that question, there are several things you must know about the fat in your food and how it relates to the fat on your body.

Which Foods Contain Fat?

Many foods contain fat: all animal products such as meat, fish, and poultry, and dairy products like butter, cream, cheese, milk, and yogurt (unless the fat has been removed such as in nonfat dairy products). Also nuts, seeds, and their oils, contain fat, as do prepared foods like mayonnaise, salad dressings, and baked goods. Breads, cereals, other whole grains, and even some fruits and vegetables also contain small amounts of fat; however, these foods are primarily composed of carbohydrates (with a few exceptions) so we do not refer to them when we refer to foods that contain fat.

A Look at Fat: The Prince Beyond the Frog

"Fatphobics" may be surprised to learn that you actually need fat in your diet (and you even need a little on your body) for good health. Fat on your body can act as a shock absorber by supporting and cushioning your organs. Without fat to do this job, you would not even be able to go horseback riding without serious injury to your internal organs. If you don't have enough fat in your diet, your skin may be very dry, scaly, and lifeless. Fatty acids also provide the raw materials that help in the control of blood pressure, blood clotting, inflammation, and other body functions.

AVOCADO, YES . . . BUT DON'T EVEN THINK ABOUT GUA-CAMOLE. Most guacamole is made from some avocado and a lot of sour cream. Limit your avocado to ¼ cup mashed.

OH, SOY! The fat from these foods is just dandy. Tofu, soy milk, soy cheeses, and other foods that come from the soybean contain primarily "friendly" fats. So stick to our portion sizes and you'll "soyly" fire up your metabolism!

LOVE FATTY DRESSING BUT WANT TO SAVE YOUR WAISTLINE? Ask that your dressing be served on the side, or if you are at home, put it on the side of your salad. Dip your fork in the dressing and stab your salad. (You can use this fork-dipping tactic for any entrée that comes with a fatty sauce on top.) You get the flavor without all the fat and calories.

Fat is essential because it helps your body to absorb the fat-soluble vitamins A, D, E, and K. These vitamins are critical for vision, normal bone and tooth growth, fertility, and boosting your immune system.

The biggest surprise of all is that fat provides long-lasting energy. As you may remember from Chapters 2 and 3, carbohydrates are the body's preferred source of energy, especially for the brain and nerve cells, and carbs provide the body with energy that is stored in the body as glycogen. But the body cannot store enough glycogen to provide energy for very long. That's where fat comes to the rescue. Fat helps to spare your stored glycogen (energy) by providing fuel.

Carbohydrates are stored in muscle as glycogen—muscle energy that the body uses as it needs it. This means that fat speeds up your metabolism by providing some fuel and helping to make carbohydrates available for a longer period of time, providing more long-lasting energy. You have the energy to be more active, which means you burn more calories through activity.

Another major function of fat, other than the taste and the texture it gives foods, is to help keep you satiated. In some respects, this makes fat similar to protein. What's more, like protein, fat eaten with carbohydrates helps your blood sugar level remain stable. That means you don't get a sugar high followed by a sugar low and an energy crash, so your brain is not signaled that you need more food shortly after you eat. If you have ever ventured to the vending machine for an afternoon snack and chosen a sugary treat like Twizzlers to give you an energy boost, then you are familiar with the energy high and low we are talking about. More than likely, you were back at the vending machine an hour later craving more food and another energy boost. Obviously, this situation can spell trouble as it causes you to overeat. Surprisingly, if you had chosen peanut M&M's, you would have been better off. We are not promoting peanut M&M's as a healthy snack (sorry to disappoint you). Nor are we suggesting adding butter to your bread or eating buttered popcorn. However, eating a small amount of fat with your carbohydrate—for example, spreading a tablespoon of peanut butter (fat) on an apple (carbohydrate), or in the case of the peanut M&M's, adding the peanuts (fat) to the sugary chocolate—gives you a more steady supply of energy, preventing you from experiencing a sugar high followed by a low and energy slump. So combining a little fat with a carbohydrate helps you to avoid eating excess food. Thank you, fat.

TIP

DON'T BE A PUTZ, CHOOSE SOY NUTS. These nuts are a great alternative to peanuts, and they offer all of the benefits of the soybean. Note: Like all nuts, they are filling and satiating, but their portion must be limited to $1/4$ cup roasted because they are calorie dense.

Fat can also provide your body with a last resort for energy. This is especially important in third world countries where hunger is common. For most of you, the likelihood of having to use fat as your last resort for energy is extremely low, as we live in a society where all

Many people want to lose weight in a hurry and try semistarvation diets, where they exist on very low-carbohydrate, low-calorie diets (fewer than one thousand calories a day). These diets cause your body to react in a way similar to fasting and can cause some initial weight loss from water and lean tissue. However, you rapidly regain the weight, and then some, when you start eating normally again. Not only does the water weight come back immediately, such diets clearly backfire as you wind up burning up muscle rather than fat; you slow your metabolism rather than rev it up.

food seems to be supersized and most people tend to fall in the "feast" rather than "famine" category. However, if you are a contestant on the television show *Survivor,* or find yourself starving for some other reason, your body would use up all of its carbohydrate stores, and then it would eat up its protein stores, burning its muscles for fuel. Then your body would rely on its savior—your body fat stores—as its last line of defense to save you from starvation, sparing you from having to completely burn up your organs and your heart for fuel.

TIPS

SUPER SEEDS! SUNFLOWER, ROASTED DRY, BUT JUST A SPRINKLE. Just two tablespoons is all it takes to add spunk to any meal. It'll keep you satisfied while firing you up.

WHAT'S BETTER THAN PEANUT BUTTER? Peanut butter is scrumptious, satisfying, and a great way to make the energy and metabolism-revving boost of the carbohydrate last longer. However, like any food high in fat, calories from peanut butter add up very quickly—so stick to one flat tablespoon.

PARMESAN CHEESE? YES, PLEASE! At only twenty-two calories per tablespoon, top salads with two tablespoons instead of calorie-dense salad dressing!

How You Can Burn Fats and How They Can Help You Fire Up Your Metabolism

So now you know that among many other benefits, fat helps to keep you satiated so that you don't overeat, and it provides more long-lasting energy so that you burn more calories. You also know that during starvation, you burn your body fat stores for energy, which is lifesaving. However, on the downside, you also know that during such a situation and while on semistarvation diets, you lose large amounts of your calorie-burning lean muscle tissue as well. So you are probably asking, "Well, what about under normal circumstances, when I'm not starving myself? Can't I burn fat for energy without eating my lean muscle tissue?"

The answer is yes, you can manipulate your body to burn fat for energy, and that takes us to another chivalrous property of fat—you can spare your protein stores (muscle) by burning fat for energy. (Now we're talking! Isn't this what we all want to do—burn fat cell after fat cell, yet keep our muscle tone?) However, there is a catch. In order to completely burn fat, you must provide your body with some carbohydrates (see Chapter 2 to see which carbohydrates, and how much of them, you should choose). It's as simple as that. If you don't have carbohydrates available to provide energy for your brain and central nervous system, fat won't be completely broken down for energy, and a dangerous condition called ketosis will set in. (Remember that ketosis is the end product of incomplete fat breakdown. It negatively affects your body's acid-base balance, leading to headache, fatigue, and nausea, and ultimately slowing your metabolism.)

TIPS

TRY SWEET PEPITAS ROASTED PUMPKIN SEEDS. They pack seven grams of fiber (more than the amount in three slices of whole wheat bread) and protein into every one-ounce serving. And they're high in zinc to help you to have a healthy immune system.

The best part? The maple syrup and pumpkin pie–spice flavored seeds have only 150 calories and eight grams of fat. They also come in spicy, extra hot spicy, and chocolate. To order, go to thefertilehand.com. Two tablespoons equal one fat serving.

CHARLIE BROWN KNEW WHAT HE WAS DOING BY JOINING THE PEANUTS. Satiating peanuts are packed with nutrients. Combine two tablespoons with 1/4 cup no-sugar-added, low-fat granola and you'll have one great snack.

ADD ZIP TO ALMOST ANY DISH. Blue Diamond Almond Toppers are not just plain old almonds. They come in flavors. We recommend adding Spicy Szechuan to stir-fries, Roasted Garlic or Country Ranch to salads or baked potatoes, and Sun-Dried Tomato and Basil or Robust Parmesan to pasta or rice. Just remember, two tablespoons equal one of your fat servings.

So now you know the good news: You need some fat in your diet and, better yet, you know that you can burn fat off your body as long as you eat some carbohydrates. However, when it comes to eating fat, there is something else you must know.

Fat Beauties and Beasts

Have you ever heard that there is one good twin and one evil one? Well, it is definitely true. Lyssie is the angel, while Tammy is the bad twin. The reason we are telling you this is that just as there is a good twin and a bad twin, there are good fats and bad fats. Similarly, all fats have good and bad characteristics, but some fats have a lot more hidden beasts.

The beauties of the fats are good for your health and helpful for your metabolism, and we refer to them as "friendly." You should continue your relationship with these fats in our specified amounts, as they can be helpful for firing up your metabolism for the rest of your life.

On the other hand, the ugly beasts of the fats can harm your health and ultimately depress your metabolism. Therefore, we call these fats "foes," and your relationship with them should end. They are beasts that weigh you down, interfere with your ability to have a fully powered metabolism, and eventually harm your health and hamper your weight-loss efforts.

Fat "Foes" and Why You Should Rarely Eat Them

The fats we call "foes" are found in butter; beef and beef fat; poultry and poultry fat; lard; dairy products made with whole milk (these are counted as "thumbs-down" proteins because of their artery-clogging *fat*), such as cheese, ice cream, and yogurt; palm oil and palm kernel oil; and hydrogenated fats found in foods like margarine, fried foods, baked goods, cookies, cakes, croissants, and many fast-food items. The medical community refers to these "foes" as saturated fats and trans fats. They are responsible for raising your body's bad cholesterol (low-density lipoproteins, LDLs) level and for making your blood "sticky." "Sticky" blood doesn't flow well through your body and has a difficult time carrying nutrients and oxygen to your muscles. Less oxygen equals less energy in a less efficiently running body.

And although no scientific studies have been performed on metabolism and the different kinds of fat, we believe that the fats we call the "foes" slow your metabolism since they cause you to have "thick and sticky" blood and clogged vessels. These "foes" create havoc as blood flow throughout your body becomes difficult. Therefore, your bodily processes, including your metabolism, are not able to perform optimally. The "foes"—saturated fats and trans fats—also increase your risk of heart disease. So to keep your blood from getting "sticky," choose the "friendly" fats, as it is evident that the "foes" hold quite a grudge after they are eaten.

TIPS

LOBSTER BISQUE? IT'S NOT WORTH THE RISK. Bisque is full of calorie- and fat-laden cream. Stay away.

SAY IT AIN'T SO! MAYONNAISE, YOU'VE GOTTA GO! Packed with five grams of saturated and trans fat and one hundred calories per tablespoon, you're much better off choosing fat-free mayonnaise dressing for ten calories per tablespoon, or choosing mustard and ketchup as condiments.

BYE-BYE BLUE CHEESE. Just two tablespoons of blue cheese salad dressing is 160 calories—that's more calories than a slice of whole wheat bread with a slice of nonfat cheese, tomato, and lettuce on it.

CREAM AND CHEESE . . . TWO THINGS THAT SHOULD NEVER BE COMBINED! Try this better bagel spread: Smear on some fromage blanc, a soft French cheese that's rich and creamy but made with skim milk so it's fat free and only fifteen calories per ounce. But check the labels—some manufacturers add cream. You can call Vermont Butter & Cheese Company (one of the biggest U.S. makers) and order direct: (800) 884-6287. Fat-free cream cheese is your other option.

How Do "Friendly" Fats Help Fire Up My Metabolism?

"Friendly" fats are found in avocados, olives, nuts, seeds, soybeans (and tofu) and their oils, as well as the oils found in fish. These fats are also called unsaturated fats, and they not only prolong the metabolic boost of the carbohydrate they are combined with, but also are good for your heart and for the rest of your body. Eating "friendly" fats instead of the "foes" can help decrease your risk of heart attack and also make your blood less "sticky." "Friendly" fats actually help to keep your blood clot-free. The "friendly" omega-3 fats that are found in fish ("always" proteins), and in smaller amounts in flaxseeds and walnuts, appear to help increase your body's good cholesterol and decrease your body's bad cholesterol while also stabilizing your heart cell membranes and making your blood less likely to clot (or, as we like to say, less "sticky"). To have an efficiently functioning body that is adequately supplied with blood and oxygen—and to fire up your metabolism—choose the "friendly" fats. (Note: Although fish contain omega-3 fatty acids, fish is still considered a protein food, so you will find fish serving sizes in the protein chapter, Chapter 4, rather than in this chapter.)

Kick Your Foes to the Curb and Replace Them with Friends

To make sure you eat the "friendly" fats, cook with olive oil instead of butter; spread peanut butter, almond butter, or hummus rather than cream cheese or butter on your whole wheat English muffin. Sprinkle sesame seeds, sunflower seeds, or nuts rather than full-fat cheese (counted as a "thumbs-down" protein because it is packed with fat) on your salad. Make sandwiches with avocado rather than with fatty meats like bologna and salami. And don't top those sandwiches with mayonnaise. Instead, try soy mayo, or choose mustard or nonfat mayo and save a fat option for another meal. Use vinaigrette dressing rather than a creamy salad dressing. Order fish rather than steak for your entrée.

Although small portions of all fats temporarily jump-start your metabolism when combined with a carbohydrate, when it comes to your long-term health and having a speedy metabolism for the rest of

You can purchase "milled" (ground) or "whole" flaxseeds (also called linseeds) at health food stores or some supermarkets in the bulk food section. If you buy them whole, use a small food processor, blender, or coffee grinder to crush them. Otherwise, the whole seeds pass through your system without being absorbed and you don't benefit from their omega-3 fatty acids. Flaxseeds in yogurt, salads, cereals, casseroles, and breads add a pleasant, nutty flavor.

your life, only the "friendly" fats are beautiful both inside and out. Just remember: Although these "friendly" fats are better than the "foes" for firing up your metabolism and for your long-term health, *all* fats ultimately lead to weight gain and depress your metabolic rate when eaten in excess. Therefore, mixing the right portions of fat with the appropriate servings of specific carbohydrates (see "always" carbohydrates in Chapter 2) is essential for a speedy metabolism. Below, you will find the number of fat servings you need each day to fire it up. The number of fat servings you must restrict yourself to each day is equal to the amount of fruit servings you need each day. (Note: There is an exception. If your level (determined on page 63 is 1,200 or 1,300, your fruit servings don't equal your fat servings.)

TIPS

NEW ENGLAND'S OUT. MANHATTAN IS IN. CLAM CHOWDER, THAT IS. New England Clam Chowder is cream based and contains more than twice as much fat and artery-clogging fat as its southern tomato-based partner.

POTATO CHIPS? ONLY IF YOU MAKE THEM YOURSELF! Preheat your oven to 400 degrees. Wash a large potato and cut it in thin slices. Spray a cooking sheet with cooking spray. Place potato slices in a single layer, spray lightly with oil, and sprinkle with paprika. Bake for thirty minutes, turning once. Slices should be crisp and brown.

JUST A DASH WILL DO. Use a dash of Mrs. Dash instead of butter or oil on veggies, baked potatoes, rice, and pastas and save hundreds of calories.

Remember, eating the right amount of fat is critical for speeding up your metabolism. Eating too little fat or too much fat results in a body fat increase and weight gain.

Daily Fat Servings

YOUR NUMBER FROM STEP 1 (See page 63)	YOUR LEVEL (To be applied in later chapters)	YOUR DAILY FAT SERVINGS
1,200	12	$\frac{1}{2}$
1,300	13	1
1,400	14	2
1,500	15	$2\frac{1}{2}$
1,600	16	$2\frac{1}{2}$
1,700	17	$2\frac{1}{2}$
1,800	18	3
1,900	19	3
2,000	20	3
2,100	21	3
2,200	22	$3\frac{1}{2}$
2,300	23	4
2,400	24	4
2,500	25	4
2,600	26	$4\frac{1}{2}$
2,700	27	$4\frac{1}{2}$
2,800	28	5
2,900	29	5
3,000–3,199	30	$5\frac{1}{2}$
3,200	31	6
3,300–3,499	32	6
3,500	33	$6\frac{1}{2}$

A Give-and-Take Relationship: When It Comes to Firing It Up, Fats Don't Work Alone

Now you know that in order to have a speedy metabolism, you must provide your body with some fats and some carbohydrates, as they help each other. As a matter of fact, when it comes to carbohydrates and fat, having one without the other results in a depressed metabolic rate. If you ate only carbohydrates and no fat, your energy boost would be short-lived and you would soon have very little energy to be active. If you ate only fats and deprived your body of carbohydrates, your body would try to burn fat for fuel yet would not be able to completely break it down (who wants the remnants of fat floating around?) and, meanwhile, your body would also eat your calorie-burning muscle for energy. Remember, "fats burn in the fire of carbohydrates," so once your carbohydrate stores are used up, you are no longer able to completely burn fat.

TIPS

SMART MOVE, POPEYE . . . LIVE FOR THE OLIVE! Olives are a "friendly" fat. However, more than several moments on the lips equals a lifetime on the hips. Black or green, stick to ¼ cup.

SEE YA, SAUSAGE! UNLESS IT'S MORNINGSTAR FARMS BREAKFAST PATTIES. Compared to two ounces of McDonald's sausage patties, just two ounces of these patties save you more than 110 calories and seventeen grams of fat, six of those artery clogging. (Other great-tasting brands of faux sausage made from soy are now available in the freezer section of your supermarket.)

If Some Fat Is Good, Is More Merrier?

Although only small quantities of fat are necessary for good health, people overindulge in fatty foods. A high-fat diet (even if it's the "friendly" fats) raises your risk of cancer. Also, since fat takes six to eight hours to digest, when you eat a large fatty meal, most of your blood rushes to your stomach for digestion and stays there for a long time, leaving your brain and muscles with inadequate blood supply and oxygen, making you feel sluggish. If you've ever sat down to a big steak dinner or a breakfast of buttery eggs, fried potatoes, and bacon, you know what we are talking about and are probably all too familiar with this "after-meal coma." Most people will admit to feeling a little hung over after Sunday brunch.

This "after-meal coma" was a feeling that Bob was all too familiar with. Bob had the best intentions of exercising every day after work. He usually ate a late lunch at 2:00, hoping it would give him energy for his 4:30 workout. His lunch was usually an extra-cheese pepperoni and sausage pizza, or a bacon cheeseburger, or tomato and mozzarella on a croissant from a local deli. He said that no matter how much he wanted to go to the gym and no matter how much sleep he had gotten the night before, by late afternoon, he felt extremely sluggish and too tired to muster up the energy to go. We pointed out that each of Bob's lunches contributed calories that were primarily from fat (and a quite large amount of it), which was causing his body to send blood and oxygen to his stomach, leaving very little for his brain and muscles, and thus the lethargy.

So we put Bob on our Fire Up Your Metabolism plan. At lunch, he made slight changes in his usual selections, but he didn't have to eat rabbit food, or forgo the foods he loved. We had him get rid of the fatty pepperoni and sausage on his pizza and order extra veggies instead. Bob also began ordering the pizza "light on the cheese" so that fat was reduced to an acceptable level. And instead of the bacon cheeseburger, he had a grilled chicken sandwich with barbeque sauce or mustard. Instead of the tomato and mozzarella on a croissant, he would choose a chicken, bean, and veggie wrap with salsa. When Bob made these changes, he was astounded: He had energy at 4:30! He was able to make late-afternoon workouts a regular routine. That's not all that became a regular routine: Dropping several pounds on the scale became a biweekly routine as well. Bob was thrilled and said his abs were finally the way he had always wanted them to be—he had sped up his metabolism and could now see a six-pack. He was shocked. "And to think that I was just about to give up the thought of ever making it to the gym!"

More Fat Is Not Merrier

Despite its few good qualities, too much fat will make you gain body fat faster than anything else because it is calorie dense. A gram of carbohydrate or protein contains only four calories. However, a gram of fat contains nine calories, more than twice as many as carbohydrates or proteins. To help you to visualize this better, think of it this way: If you take a bite of a carbohydrate food or a bite of a protein food and compare it to an equal-size bite of a fat food, the food composed of fat would have more than twice as many calories as the same-size bite of the carbohydrate or protein food.

You may be asking, "What does that mean for me?" Well, it means that when you consume fat, it is easy to consume excess calories. Eating more calories than your body requires causes you to gain weight; eating fewer calories and/or exercising more than your body requires in order to maintain its weight causes you to lose weight.

Not only is it easy to consume excess calories from fatty foods, you also are more likely to gain weight if your excess calories come from fatty foods. When you overeat calories from protein or carbohydrates, your body must first process them and put them through a lot of transformations before it can store them as fat. On the other hand, when you eat excess calories from fat, your body recognizes it as fat and can store it directly without having to put it through any conversions. So eating a fatty food creates a weight gain issue that is double trouble. If you indulge in fatty foods like creamy sauces and fatty meats, you consume excess calories that are very easily stored as fat.

TIPS

DITCH THE MARGARINE AND THE BUTTER, WE'VE GOT SOMETHING BETTER. Try I Can't Believe It's Not Butter *spray*. It's calorie-free, fat-free, and sodium-free . . . and it's got tons of taste. You *really* won't believe it's not butter! Use the spray (not tub) on your morning toast instead of butter and lose ½ pound per week.

COOKING IN OIL? TRY A SPRAY, A MUCH BETTER WAY! Put your favorite oil for cooking in a spray bottle and spray one to two sprays on your pan. It keeps the calories to a minimum by preventing the dumping-oil-in-the-pan syndrome. Do the same for slaw, salad, and veggie recipes that call for a bit of oil. Just spray your favorite oil on them rather than drenching them.

REDUCED-FAT PEANUT BUTTER IS NOT BETTER THAN FULL-FAT PEANUT BUTTER. Full-fat peanut butter has sixteen grams of mainly heart-healthy fat in two tablespoons, while reduced-fat peanut butter has twelve grams. However, the calories in both are practically the same, thanks to the cornstarch and other fillers added to the reduced-fat version.

TWO PERCENT MILK IS NOT MUCH BETTER THAN WHOLE MILK. Whole milk is 3 percent fat. So choose 1 percent or skim milk, which are much better.

Clients Who Have Made Big, FAT Mistakes

Dorothy came to us after she had unsuccessfully tried to lose weight by dieting. She had abandoned the bread on her turkey sandwich at lunch, eating only the plain turkey and replacing the bread with a vegetable salad, as she had assumed that the bread from the sandwich would thwart her efforts to lose weight. Dorothy was discouraged—not only had she not lost any weight, she actually had packed on four pounds after starting her diet four months ago. Dorothy assumed that eating a vegetable salad rather than bread would save her two hundred calories. Her salad contained only about fifty calories, consisting of about two cups of lettuce with vegetables. However, this was before adding the dressing. Dorothy insisted that her salad dressing (vinegar and oil) was just a "sprinkle's worth." We asked Dorothy to measure exactly how much olive oil she was typically drizzling on her salad. After measuring, Dorothy reported back to us, "I knew I wasn't using much, just four tablespoons of oil."

Little did Dorothy realize that the oil she "sprinkled" on her salad was adding a hefty 480 calories! Dropping this oil from her salad would promote a weight loss of one pound per week. We had Dorothy flavor her salad with balsamic *vinegar* (*not* balsamic vinaigrette) and one teaspoon of sunflower seeds while making several other small dietary changes. It is no surprise that she has lost twenty-five pounds and has kept them off for two years and counting! (Don't worry about calculating the amount of calories your body needs to fire up your metabolism. Follow our tips and the work is done for you.)

So some fat is good, but more is not better. Just as carbohydrates and proteins need to be eaten in specific portions, the same is true for fat. Therefore, if you stick to our specified portions of fats, you will fire up your metabolism. Fat prolongs the energy and metabolic boost of carbohydrates, enabling you to have more sustained energy, be more active, and burn more calories all day long. In addition, fat keeps you satiated, preventing you from bingeing and overeating at your next meal.

TIPS

THROW OUT THOSE "FAT-FREE" POTATO CHIPS MADE WITH "FAKE FAT." These chips are made with a fat substitute called Olestra. Olestra, for some, is a laxative and sends them sprinting to the bathroom with terrible stomach pains. It is not absorbed and passes through the body—on its way out, it pulls important fat-soluble vitamins A, D, E, and K and also carotenoids. In fact, the role of fat-soluble nutrients is so valuable that we would rather have you eat the real potato chips than this "rarely" carbohydrate potato chip made with Olestra.

DON'T GET BURNED BY FAT-BURNER SUPPLEMENTS. Supplements like Fat-Trapper, CitraLean, and Ultra Burn have never been proven effective. Save your pennies, or maybe we should say hundreds of dollars. Burning a hole in your pocket is all these supplements do.

WHAT DO FISH OIL SUPPLEMENTS LACK? FISH OIL. According to *Tufts University Health and Nutrition Letter,* people who take supplements (which are supposed to be much richer in fish oil than the fish itself) in hopes of gaining a healthier heart may be in for a disappointment. A third of the brands tested fell short anywhere from 18–67 percent of the two omega-3 fatty acids that they claimed they contained. Not to mention, a daily dosage of the average fish oil tablets adds about fifty calories to your daily caloric intake—this is more than five pounds over the course of a year.

Our Twin Trial

in which you see that not all fats are your enemy

When it came time to do the twin trial for fat, deciding what specific trial to conduct was a real challenge, as fat affects your metabolism and your weight in myriad ways. We thought about testing fat's ability to extend the energy boost of carbohydrates and show how—when eaten in specific portions—it provides longer-lasting energy and allows for more activity and for more calories to be burned, while also stabilizing blood sugar levels and preventing sugar highs and crashes and the subsequent cravings and overeating.

However, since proteins have this same ability, we rejected this idea; many people already realize how hungry they feel shortly after eating a carbohydrate by itself (without some fat or protein) and that their energy is short-lived. Think about how soon you feel hungry after eating just a slice of toast for breakfast.

So we decided to test fat in two other ways, and this time we were both losers. That's right, the coin flip didn't determine who won and who lost; instead, it determined which guinea pig trial we each would take part in. For three months, Tammy was to go on a high-fat diet, hoping to show how just choosing too many fatty foods can really affect weight. Although Tammy's trial was looking at the effect of fatty foods on body weight and body fat percentage, rather than on metabolism, we felt it was important to include this trial because, even though it sounds obvious, most people just don't seem to realize how much eating fatty foods can hinder their weight-loss efforts. As we noted before, carbohydrates have become a culprit, and people are confused about fats; when they hear that a fat is healthy, they think that it won't affect their weight and they are even more bewildered. So we wanted to prove just how detrimental overeating fats can be— and to show stark results so that there would never be a question about fat. We knew very well what the results of this trial would be, and that is why neither of us jumped to do it. However, when it came to the other trial, we both were even less enthusiastic. Lyssie had to do the worse of the two evils; she had to choose the fat "foes" rather than the "friendly" fats, which are downright detrimental to your health, and just the thought of it made us cringe.

Tammy: My job in the study was to replace all of the low- and nonfat foods I regularly eat with their healthy yet high-fat counterparts. For example, my average breakfast of one cup All-Bran extra-fiber cereal with ³/₄ cup low-fat soy milk and an apple was to be changed to the high-fat version. So the ³/₄ cup low-fat soy milk was replaced with ³/₄ cup regular soy milk. In addition, instead of eating other heart-healthy, low-fat foods, I ate their high-fat counterparts: full-fat soy yogurt replaced nonfat yogurt; I used oil instead of cooking spray; leaner meats and fishes such as haddock, tuna, and swordfish gave way to fatty fishes like salmon, herring, and sardines. Fat-free and low-fat dressings, mayonnaise, and sauces were replaced with high-fat versions. For example, instead of seasoning my tuna (canned in water) sandwiches with nonfat mayonnaise, lemon, and pepper, or mustard, I used regular, full-fat Nayonnaise (heart-healthy soy-based mayo) or tuna canned in oil. And instead of using balsamic vinegar or nonfat dressings on my salads, I had full-fat oil dressings and vinaigrette dressings; at restaurants, I ordered salads without requesting the dressing on the side, so that the dressing was already on the salad when I received it. In addition, I chose garlic and oil sauces over wine, tomato-based, lemon, and plain garlic sauces, and I ate fish and meats sautéed in olive oil rather than grilled.

Guess what? This trial was easy and enjoyable. I loved the foods.

Meats cooked in olive oil had a nice flavor, as did the regular soy milk, and the vinaigrette dressings gave salads a new zing. I felt satiated because I was allowed to eat my usual "always" carbohydrates with the healthy full-fat foods.

And I felt great. I had tons of energy and never once felt hungry. Best of all, I didn't feel guilty about enjoying this meal plan, because I was choosing heart-healthy fats in moderate portions, which wouldn't sabotage my health.

There was a bad side, though. I didn't like what I saw in the mirror. After seventeen days, I started to see slight bulges in places I had never seen them before—the sides of my upper thighs and the front of my lower stomach. This is what I had expected, but actually having to deal with it and the discomfort of tight pants was annoying and uncomfortable.

I am grateful to Lyssie for agreeing that I could do the trial for four weeks instead of three months. After four weeks, when it was time to measure my body fat, the results were just as we had expected, and I was not happy. The calories from fat, even the heart-healthy kind, still add up quickly and greatly affect weight and body fat percentage. My body fat had increased 5.1 percent and I had gained 5½ pounds during the four weeks! Despite enjoying the foods I ate, they weren't worth the body changes I experienced.

Looking back, I still I can't believe that I felt so healthy and energetic even though my clothes felt as though they had shrunk a size in the dryer.

Unfortunately, I had a surprising reaction when I returned to my old Fire Up Your Metabolism habits: I no longer enjoyed the taste of the low-fat foods. Considering the effects of the higher-fat diet on my metabolism, I knew I had to return to my old ways. So for fourteen days I returned to my pretrial nonfat and low-fat foods, even though they weren't as delicious as what I had been eating. Then, surprisingly, my taste buds adjusted. The lesson learned: If you don't like the low-fat or nonfat good-for-your-metabolism foods, be patient and stick it out for two to three weeks. Soon your taste buds will turn over, like all cells in your body, and adjust to the new flavor, and you will appreciate these healthy foods.

Lyssie: I agreed to eat the fat "foes" instead of the "friendly" fats, testing our hypothesis that the "foes," which are responsible for raising the body's bad cholesterol levels and making the blood "sticky," ultimately slow the metabolism.

We had my cholesterol measured before and after the three-month trial; an increase in cholesterol would signify that my blood vessels were more susceptible to forming plaque and my blood was more susceptible to becoming "sticky," therefore making blood flow throughout the body more difficult. If blood and oxygen supply becomes restricted, even slightly, the body runs less efficiently, and all processes, including metabolism, are affected.

Although this hypothesis has not been scientifically tested, we believe the metabolism-slowing effects seen from choosing the fat "foes" are magnified as time passes, as damage from saturated and trans fat accumulates. So although this trial would last only three months, the harm to the body, and to the metabolism, would worsen with every passing month if I regularly continued to choose the "foes."

This trial took quite a bit of planning. We realized that the effects on metabolism and body fat from eating fat "foes" for several months would be much less significant than the effects of regularly eating the "foes" for a lifetime. Since I eat just several fat servings (all "friendly") a day, we didn't expect to see immediate changes in my cholesterol and/or metabolism if I just replaced those few fat servings with the fat "foes" for the duration of this short trial. So we added several more fat servings each day than I usually eat while removing all "friendly" fats. The trickiest part was that we had to be sure that I was not eating more calories than I usually do, as that would affect my body fat level. It took work, but we managed to subtract calories elsewhere. For instance, my treats, like frozen yogurt, were eliminated so that butter or mayo could be added to my menu.

To this day, I insist that the no-frozen-yogurt rule was the toughest part of the trial.

So I avoided my usual "friendly" fats like peanut butter, olive oil, hummus, almonds, homemade granola made with nuts and seeds, and canola and safflower oils. I threw out a carton of nonfat frozen yogurt so that I would not be tempted. I ate only saturated, artery-clogging, fat-laden butter, mayo, full-fat dairy products, creamy sauces, and salad dressings, as well as fatty meats like bacon and fatty cuts of steak (fish was not allowed), and fried foods.

For the first couple of weeks of the diet, some of the adjustments were difficult. Forcing myself to drink whole milk rather than soy milk in my cereal was nearly impossible in the beginning—it seemed as though I was drinking cream. I frequently felt sick, especially after eating at restaurants, as my stomach was not accustomed to all the heavy, fatty foods. Cream sauces and fried meats seemed to cause the most problems.

I know you're not really feeling sorry for me. I will admit that after eighteen days, I began to enjoy the flavor of the fatty foods. If I didn't have to sit there with a pen and add up my daily calories to make sure that I wasn't eating more than usual, I would have had a really good time. So to make life easier, I started to have "usual" meals, just so I wouldn't have to calculate my daily calories. Breakfast was either whole milk and cereal or a slice of whole wheat toast and a few slices of bacon. Instead of eating nonfat cheese or tuna on bread at lunch, I started having the equivalent in calories of butter on bread. And I replaced lean fish or chicken breast for dinner with the same calorie portion of fried fish, steak, or full-fat cheese. Once it became routine, it was easy and tasty.

The downside was that the diet changes started to take a toll on my body immediately after the completion of my meals. These fatty foods seemed to sit in my stomach; they took a long time to digest, and they made me feel tired. For several hours, I didn't feel much like doing anything but sitting still and waiting for my food to digest. I felt as though the fatty foods were weighing me down. Ironically, we later found out that is exactly what the fatty foods did.

At the end of the trial, I was relieved that I didn't really notice any difference in my overall mood and energy level, aside from feeling sluggish for a few hours after completing my meals. But it was time to check the less-visible effects. My low-density lipoprotein (bad) cholesterol level, which was 89 mg/dL at the start of the trial, now was 97 mg/dL, which surprised us. Although I was still within the American Heart Association recommendations (it is desirable to keep your LDL cholesterol level below 130 and optimal to keep it below 100 mg/dL), we had not expected to see my bad cholesterol go up more than a point or two, if at all. This trial was only three months long; I had a lifetime of good eating habits under my belt, and I was still eating my usual healthy foods, like beans, oats, fruits, and vegetables—all of which contain soluble fiber and help to keep bad cholesterol levels down. However, maybe this rise in my LDL cholesterol level occurred not only because I added the artery clogging "foes" to my diet but also because I was not eating the usual "friendly" fats, particularly the polyunsaturated fats (found in corn, safflower, and soybean oils [tofu, soymilk, etc.] and cold-water fish) that lower LDL cholesterol when used to replace saturated fats.

Just before I was weighed and had my body fat level tested, I said that I was relieved that I didn't notice any changes in my body or in my muscle tone and was glad that I had meticulously measured portion sizes of the "foes" to ensure that I did not consume more calories while on the trial. However, despite what I believed, the results revealed that I had gained one pound and my body fat was 0.8 percent higher. We both were quite surprised by this; we did not expect that the fat "foes" were capable of doing their dirty deed in just three months.

There are two possible reasons for this increase in body fat. First, maybe the fatty meals that were making me sluggish were causing me to be less active during the course of the day, thereby causing me to burn fewer calories and thus slowing my metabolism. Or possibly the "foes," which are responsible for raising your LDL cholesterol, were causing the blood to become more "sticky" and therefore hampering blood flow throughout the body. If blood and oxygen supply becomes restricted even slightly, the body runs less efficiently, and all processes, including the metabolism, are affected. Whether the increase in body fat was due to a slowdown in metabolism from one or both of these possibilities, we were shocked to see that the metabolism was affected in such a short time. This convinces us that choosing the "friendly" fats rather than the "foes" is even more critical for firing up your metabolism than we previously thought.

KISS QUICHE GOOD-BYE. Just one-eighth of a pie has five hundred calories, forty-eight grams of fat (more than half a day's worth for most people), twenty-eight grams of saturated fat (more than a day's worth), and 285 milligrams of cholesterol (about a day's worth). The culprits for these high numbers are the pie crust, eggs, cream, and cheese.

**THINKING ABOUT A STARBUCKS TWENTY-OUNCE MOCHA COF-
FEE DRINK? THINK AGAIN.** Made with fatty whole milk and
whipped cream, this drink will give you 510 calories—almost a
third of the calories that many women need in their entire day. And
this is before you even eat!

**AND FRAPPUCCINO . . . WHO WOULD THINK IT COULD FRUMP
YOU UP?** Who knew that Starbucks's lowest-calorie and lowest-
saturated-fat frappuccino would be their original venti coffee frappuccino with four hundred calories and eighteen teaspoons of
sugar? But don't keel over yet. They now offer other frappuccino
options that range from 600 to 870 calories and up to thirty-two
grams of bad fat. This is almost three-quarters of the calories some
of you may need in a day, and this comes before you even eat anything.

ONE TIME YOU SHOULDN'T EAT YOUR CAKE AND HAVE IT TOO.
Carrot cake is packed with artery-clogging fat and will give you
more than thirteen hundred calories. Although it sounds healthy,
carrot cake is actually quite the opposite. It's made from two
"foes," sour cream and cream cheese.

FORGO FATTY FRENCH FRIES FOR AN ENHANCED SEX LIFE. Down-
ing this high-fat food leads to clogged arteries, which makes it
harder for blood to circulate to all parts of your body, including
below the belt.

SIX

Banishing Breakfast? Beware

Myth Busters

MYTH: If you want to reap the full benefits of breakfast, you should have a traditional, large breakfast.

BUSTED: You don't have to sit down to typical, traditional breakfasts in order to be healthy. Even nontraditional breakfasts, such as a turkey breast sandwich on whole wheat bread with mustard, lettuce, and tomato, and a piece of fruit will start your morning off right. Healthy foods are healthy no matter when you eat them.

MYTH: Skipping breakfast will help you to lose weight because you will be eating less food.

BUSTED: Research shows that people who eat breakfast lose weight and keep it off most easily. Breakfast skippers seem to eat extra calories later in the day. What's more, they mess up their metabolism, which also causes them to pack on the pounds.

MYTH: Avoid eggs because they are too high in cholesterol.

BUSTED: Eggs are a great source of protein and can be part of a healthy breakfast. If you are watching your cholesterol level, simply choose Egg Beaters or egg whites, or limit your yolks to two or three per week.

Befriending Breakfast

You may have heard that breakfast is the most important meal of the day. We prefer not to slight any meals (we like them all). However, if we had to choose one as the most important, we would choose breakfast. And, as hard as it is to admit, yet again Mom was right when she told us to eat a good breakfast; it is easy to take her advice when you know it will fire up your metabolism, helping you to burn more fat and more calories all day long.

When you sleep, your body realizes that it is at rest. You digest food and burn calories more slowly. Your body, the genius that it is, takes advantage of this time to focus on healing and repairing itself from daily damages.

As your peaceful slumber continues, your body starts to feel threatened. After all, it hasn't received food in a while. Should it prepare for a fast? Taking all possible measures to keep you alive, and anticipating starvation, your body starts to conserve fuel, burning fat and calories even more slowly. So by the time you wake up in the morning, your body is in "conservation mode," reserving its energy while burning fat and calories at a slower rate.

Our Twin Trial

in which we prove that skipping breakfast slows your metabolism

Tammy: I lost the "guinea pig" coin toss and was forced to forgo breakfast for a *full two months!* I kissed Mom's granola good-bye and pushed it to the back of the cupboard, along with my boxed soy milk and my apple. I also had to give up my midmorning snack—Dannon Light N' Fit yogurt would no longer be a part of my daily routine. We decided that I was to give up both my breakfast and my midmorning snack, and just eat lunch, as the average "breakfast banisher" does. This way, I would have similar experiences to other people who skip breakfast.

Breaking my morning breakfast and midmorning ritual was torturous for eleven days. Then, strangely, it became quite easy. Finally, a trial that was painless after a little over a week—I really lucked out by getting this trial and I secretly began to celebrate. After all, I doubted that I would see any negative consequences after two months by cutting out two meals. In fact, for some reason, despite knowing that my metabolism would probably slow, I was pretty convinced that if anything were to happen, my body fat would decrease. The rumbling and grumbling of my empty stomach that had embarrassed me on the subway and had disrupted my concentration during the first eleven days was suddenly nonexistent. Even hunger pangs that I occasionally felt around 11 A.M. had completely subsided by the end of the first month. In fact, by the end of two months, I didn't *seem* to notice any negative physical effects from skipping breakfast. Little did I know that I was in for a rude awakening.

I stepped confidently on the scale, *knowing* that I would weigh the same, or perhaps even less than when the trial had begun. And although for the trial's sake I wanted to show an increase in body fat to prove what the research already shows (skipping breakfast leads to weight gain and a slowed metabolism), it was nice to know that I didn't have to compromise my body this time.

I was wrong. My body fat increased by 2.9 percent and I gained more than three pounds. I was so shocked that I remeasured, reweighed, remeasured, and reweighed. First of all, how could I not have realized that I had gained weight? And how did I not realize that my pants were tighter? (I have learned that I was so convinced I hadn't gained weight that I didn't pay attention to the way my clothes fit. This just goes to show you the power of mind over body—but that's another book.)

Second, how did my body fat increase so much in two months, despite completing my normal amount of daily exercise? The unbelievable part was that I was eating less food than I normally do. Sure, I was starving by lunch and put a little bit more tuna, turkey, or cheese on my sandwich, and maybe I had a bit more chopped fruit at lunch, but it wasn't more than what I normally ate. After all, I was cutting out an entire meal and a snack!

Even if I had added enough extra food to my lunch to make it equal in calories to what I normally ate for my breakfast and mid-morning snack, it was evident that my metabolism had slowed, since nothing else could explain the weight gain and increase in body fat. By skipping breakfast, my body must have been moving in slow gear, burning fewer calories and less fat all day, and then my body must have been overwhelmed by a slightly larger lunch than usual.

After those first eleven days, I hadn't noticed any unpleasant effects of skipping my two morning meals, so I was surprised when I did notice how much better I felt when I returned to my normal breakfast routine. I felt rejuvenated and refreshed and my lunch felt much more satiating than when I skipped breakfast.

Perhaps the most astonishing result of this trial is that Lyssie actually ate more food and calories than I did (she ate as we usually do), yet her body fat percentage did not increase.

I Thought Skipping Breakfast Helped Me Lose Weight

Many people make the critical mistake of banishing breakfast because they don't "feel hungry" in the morning and assume that they can take advantage of this time to save calories. But as you witnessed in our twin trial, skipping breakfast is troublesome.

If you don't provide your body with food (fuel) within an hour of waking up, your body remains in the "conservation mode," burning fat and calories very slowly. Clearly, this wreaks havoc on the breakfast banisher's metabolism for the rest of the day. What's more, forgoing breakfast also means that you are missing out on diet-induced thermogenesis. (You may remember from Chapter 3, diet-induced thermogenesis is the burning of calories to digest, absorb, transport, metabolize, and store ingested nutrients.) So when you eat breakfast, the calorie-burning process of diet-induced thermogenesis can begin. Countless studies show that people who regularly eat breakfast are most successful at losing weight—*and keeping it off.*

Some of the most widely publicized studies are conducted by diet researchers at the University of Colorado, the University of Pittsburgh, and Brown University, where researchers routinely collect diet data on a group of people in the National Weight Control Registry. The registry looks at people who have lost thirty pounds or more and have kept it off for a year or more. On average, these study participants had lost seventy-one pounds and kept the weight off for six years, and all participants had one thing in common: Nearly 80 percent of them ate breakfast seven days a week, and 90 percent ate breakfast at least four to six times a week.

TIPS

SMOKE IT AND SPREAD IT, AND YOU'VE GOT ONE FINE BREAKFAST. Take one ounce of smoked salmon (lox) and spread nonfat ricotta on half a whole wheat bagel. If you can't find a whole wheat bagel, use this ricotta cheese and lox topping on any other "always" carbohydrate.

OH, JUST STUFF IT! That is, half a cantaloupe with $1/2$ cup nonfat cottage cheese and a dash of cinnamon.

A TASTE OF THE MIDEAST FOR BREAKFAST. A whole wheat pita topped with three flat tablespoons of hummus.

BREAKFAST FOOD ONLY FOR BREAKFAST . . . NONSENSE! Remember, healthy foods are healthy no matter what time of day. Try a tuna fish sandwich on whole wheat bread with lettuce, tomato, and mustard, or a minipizza using a whole wheat English muffin, tomato sauce, veggies, and nonfat or low-fat cheese.

SEARCHING FOR QUAKER HARVEST CRUNCH WITH RED BERRIES? DON'T. Good thing it's a little hard to find. It's got more than six grams of fat per fifty-gram bowl.

BUCKWHEAT PANCAKES AND MAPLE SYRUP? Only if the maple syrup is *light* and limited to two tablespoons.

YOU'LL FORGET THAT THIS BREAKFAST IS HEALTHY! In a blender, combine 1 cup nonfat skim milk, 1 banana (best if frozen whole or in slices), and 1 teaspoon vanilla. While the mixture is blending, add 1 flat tablespoon of peanut butter.

What Happens Later in the Day When I Skip Breakfast

You set yourself up for the kill.

People who skip breakfast tend to select more calorie-dense foods later in the day than those who regularly eat breakfast. If you wait several hours before eating your first meal of the day, your brain will be craving fuel, and you will feel ravenous. This makes it very hard to be rational, and often poor food choices are the result. When you feel famished it is easy to overeat.

Although your body is happy to be fed, and diet-induced thermogenesis begins, eating excess food when your body is conserving fuel overwhelms your body and it stores extra calories as fat. Unfortunately, after eating this "next meal," you feel sluggish, as all of the blood leaves the brain, muscles, and other organs to rush to the stomach to aid digestion of a meal that has "overwhelmed your system." (We are all too familiar with those after-meal energy slumps that leave our already metabolically challenged bodies craving a nap and motionless—burning even fewer calories.)

The scenario we just described is what happened to Brad. He was a breakfast banisher. He claimed that he didn't feel hungry in the morning so he didn't want to waste calories eating when he didn't have an appetite. He said that an hour or so before lunchtime, he would grow quite hungry, but he forced himself to wait until lunch to eat something. Brad then would eat large portions at lunch because he was starving.

We immediately started Brad on our Fire Up Your Metabolism plan. He was skeptical and thought that eating another meal would make him gain weight. But he started by eating a small breakfast—just a slice of whole wheat toast wrapped around low-fat string cheese. (If 's stomach wasn't able to handle this much food, he could have ust a piece of fruit.) He said he couldn't believe how much more energetic he felt during the morning. Brad was finally giving his brain and muscles the fuel they needed to be active and to energize him for the start of his day. What's more, he kick-started his metabolism by allowing diet-induced thermogenesis to begin. Brad reported that at lunchtime he felt much less hungry and much more rational—and he had no problem eating a little bit smaller lunch and a healthier one. Needless to say, Brad immediately fired up his metabolism and lost seven pounds in three weeks while also stumbling upon energy in the morning.

TIPS

GO NUTS AT BREAKFAST. Try a sliced apple and a slice of whole wheat bread with one flat tablespoon of almond butter on each.

POPTARTS . . . NOT IN THIS LIFETIME. Look at the sugar and fat in this "rarely" carbohydrate and you'll know why it should be "rarely" chosen.

SPEEDY, SUPER, AND SNAZZY WAKE-UP SMOOTHIE. This is one smoothie you should actually have. Blend ¹/₂ cup frozen fruit (banana, pineapple, or peach), 1 cup nonfat light fruit-flavored yogurt, and ¹/₄ cup orange juice. You'll get fiber, an "always" carbohydrate, and a "thumbs-up" protein.

A BREAKFAST BAR FOR BREAKFAST? THINK AGAIN. This isn't a good choice. Most are loaded with sugar, and they usually have too much fat and no fiber.

BREAKFAST IN HAWAII . . . HERE'S HOW TO FAKE IT. Combine ¹/₃ cup low-fat ricotta cheese, ¹/₂ cup crushed pineapple, and a dash of nutmeg. Spread this mixture on half a whole wheat English muffin or half a small whole wheat bagel (if the first ingredient listed is whole wheat). You'll get one "always" carbohydrate, one "thumbs-up" protein, and one fruit serving.

Do You Currently Ban Breakfast?

If you currently ban breakfast, there is no need to panic. In fact, you should celebrate, as you can immediately jump-start your metabolism by eating breakfast! However, there is no need to start eating a large breakfast. Your body is not accustomed to having anything in the morning. Therefore, eating a large breakfast would be overwhelming, and although you would fire up your metabolism, you would also wind up storing some of the calories.

For now, if you have been living life as a breakfast banisher, your new breakfast will be simple: a small piece of fruit and a glass of water, which you should be able to tolerate even if the thought of food in the morning turns you off. This breakfast will allow your body to realize that it no longer needs to conserve fat and calories, and it will not be an overwhelming amount of food.

Some people make the mistake of relying solely on coffee for their morning pick-me-up, and they omit breakfast, believing that this caffeine boost is the kick their body needs. Although coffee may provide an energy boost and may—temporarily—slightly increase your metabolic rate, it actually masks the fact that the body wants (and *needs*) food to start burning calories efficiently. Many coffee-drinking, breakfast-skipping individuals are out of touch with their body's natural cry for fuel. They may trick themselves into believing they don't need fuel, but they certainly don't trick their metabolisms. Since the metabolic boost from the caffeine is slight and short-lived, forgoing food and drinking only a cup of coffee is not enough for the body to feel as though it has received fuel and it can speed up, so the body continues to conserve, burning fat and calories at a very slow rate, until it receives "real" fuel. Meanwhile, cravings for simple sugars like M&M's are inevitable as the brain is crying for a quick pick-me-up.

DO YOU LIKE SKIM LATTES? This drink actually provides enough calories for the body to feel as if it has received fuel, helping it to speed up and burn calories and fat. On the other hand, even though a frappuccino (and the caffé mocha) will allow the body to feel as if it has been fed, this beverage will overwhelm your body with 870 calories and twenty-three grams of fat.

Making Two Smart Starts: Eating Breakfast and Choosing the Right Food

What you eat for breakfast is as important as actually eating breakfast. If you make a poor choice when it comes to breakfast food, your body will avoid sensing starvation, but you still *could* gain weight.

Let's take a look at why choosing the wrong food and/or too much food at breakfast can add body fat. Let's say you have a very large (about half of your total daily food servings) or very fatty breakfast (like bacon and cheese on a large buttered biscuit—the wrong food, as discussed in Chapter 5). After the meal, your body says, "Hip-hip-hooray! I am getting food and I am not going to starve to death. I can stop conserving and start burning calories and fat." However, your body *also* says, "Hey, I am happy to be fed, but what the heck am I supposed to do with all of this food and all of these calories? This is way too much. I no longer need to conserve, but I am not going to be able to burn up all of this food either." So your body has no choice but to store some of this excess food as fat.

YOGURT—BUT NOT THE FULL-FAT VERSION. Full-fat yogurt is too high in fat (half of its calories come from fat), and too much of that fat is saturated.

ORDERING EGGS AT A DELI OR RESTAURANT? Be sure to request that cooking spray be used in the pan. Butter or oil adds hundreds of calories.

PASTRY PRUDE? IF YOU ARE, YOU'RE ONE SMART COOKIE! Most pastries are about 50 percent fat.

ORDERING AN OMELET? Make it cheeseless and save your arteries, your waistline, and your metabolism from going into overdrive. Instead, add spinach and mushrooms for a tasty alternative.

DUMP MUFFINS—EVEN THE BRAN ONES MUFF UP THE METABOLISM! They're way too fatty and filled with sugar. Bran muffins sound healthy but are also high in fat and sugar and get just a sprinkle of bran, not enough to give you its metabolism-boosting power.

WHAT'S THE WORD ON LOW-FAT MUFFINS? They're better than full fat. But you're still getting about 250 to 300 calories and close to five of your daily carbohydrate servings. So if your muffin is a must, save half for later.

CRAVING A MUFFIN? Make your own healthy version. Try an All-Bran original muffin by following the recipe on the box to pack some fiber into a much healthier muffin.

Another Typical Breakfast Mistake

You don't give your body carbohydrates. For example, you eat just a fried egg for breakfast. This is better than no breakfast at all, but it is not your best choice for firing up your metabolism. The good news is that diet-induced thermogenesis can begin. The bad news is that when you don't give your body carbohydrates, the fuel it wants to burn for energy, your body is forced to use an alternative fuel (some protein and a little fat) for energy. And that makes you tired.

On the other hand, let's say you are like Jeff and you give your body only sugary breakfast treats of simple carbohydrates or carbohydrates with no fiber, such as a fat-free muffin or Cream of Wheat. Many clients admit to having a plain, unbuttered bagel or white toast for breakfast. We applaud them for avoiding butter on their toast, for providing their body with an energy-providing carbohydrate, and for providing their body with food (and allowing the calorie-burning process of diet-induced thermogenesis to begin).

Then we must break some bad news: It is not a good idea to eat just a simple carbohydrate or a carbohydrate that doesn't have fiber in it for breakfast (or any time, for that matter). A carbohydrate with no fiber in it, like white bread, does give your body the fuel it is looking for. However, since the body wants to burn up carbohydrates so quickly, its natural response is to do just that. Your body responds to a carbohydrate with no fiber in it, by quickly digesting it and releasing glucose (blood fuel) into the blood. Your body's natural, normal, and healthy response is to release a surge of insulin, which takes the glucose from the blood to the muscles and tissues so that you can have energy. Since the glucose from the white toast was released into your bloodstream quickly and then rapidly shuttled off to your muscles, your blood will tell your brain that it needs more glucose. This is bad news, as your brain responds by making you want more food.

TIP

DITCH THE CREAM OF WHEAT—GO FOR THE OATMEAL. Oatmeal contains the whole grain. Cream of Wheat will leave you raiding the vending machine in an hour, while the oatmeal will fire up your metabolism without leaving you ravenous.

When you eat carbohydrates that contain fiber, your body gets a gradual release of glucose, providing a constant fuel source and continuing the calorie-burning process of diet-induced thermogenesis for a longer period of time. This way the brain never gets that urgent signal that it needs more food. You also avoid the sudden energy slump and hunger by combining a fibrous "always" carbohydrate (or any carbohydrate, for that matter) with a little bit of protein or fat, as discussed in Chapters 2 to 5.

WHAT A WAFFLE! THAT IS, IF IT IS WHOLE WHEAT. Packed with fiber and nutrients from the whole grain, waffles can make a great metabolism-boosting breakfast. Top them with $1/2$ cup nonfat vanilla light yogurt and $1/2$ cup fresh berries.

WHAT WAFFLE SHOULD YOU NEVER HAVE? A Belgian waffle. It's made with whole milk, eggs, butter, and a whipped topping that will weigh you down with nine hundred calories for a 7" waffle.

HOPE YOU'RE A FAN OF RAISIN BRAN! Whole grains, fruit, fiber, vitamins, and minerals all in one package! Limit cereal to $1 1/2$ cups and top with skim or low-fat milk, and this energy-boosting breakfast is sure to fire up your metabolism!

TIRED OF PLAIN OLD OATMEAL? Use quick oats and prepare according to directions in a microwave or on the stovetop. Replace water with 1 percent or skim milk. Add vanilla extract and fresh or frozen blueberries.

Choosing the Right Foods for Breakfast

We call the breakfast foods that you should choose the "always" foods (as described in Chapters 2 to 5, and listed in the "always" carbohydrates, "thumbs-up" proteins, and "friendly" fats lists). If you don't overeat these foods (no more than one-third of your total daily food servings at breakfast), you will boost your metabolism and lose fat.

STIR 1–2 TABLESPOONS SLIVERED ALMONDS into 1 cup oatmeal.

SOUP FOR BREAKFAST? It's worth a try, especially in the winter. Add tofu or chicken breast to your basic vegetable-based soup.

TOMATO CHEESE MELT. Two slices of whole wheat bread topped with tomato and $3/4$ ounce low- or nonfat cheese on each slice.

YOGURT STIR-IN. Stir $1/4$ cup no-sugar-added, low-fat granola into 1 cup nonfat, sugar-free yogurt.

ROLL AND RUN. Roll a scrambled egg (cooked in cooking spray or in a nonstick pan) and salsa into a small whole wheat tortilla.

If You're a Breakfast Banner, Here's What You Should Do

If you skip an occasional breakfast when you are in a rush, or you forget breakfast now and then, the following advice does not apply to you. But try *never* to put yourself in a situation where you must skip breakfast. Make breakfast a priority, and don't use not having enough time as an excuse—you can, at the very least, always grab a piece of fruit, nature's original fast food, on the way out the door. It's much better than eating nothing, especially when it comes to burning more fat all day long!

PREP THE NIGHT BEFORE. If you complain that you have no time in the morning, throw cereal in a bowl the night before or toss cereal in a Ziploc bag, then mix it into a container of yogurt in the morning. Or spread a tablespoon of peanut butter on bread to be wrapped around a banana.

Starting to Eat Breakfast:
Slow and Steady Wins the Metabolism Race

The process of starting to eat breakfast must be done gradually. In fact, the first day that you break free from being a habitual breakfast banner, your breakfast should be quite small, and it should continue to be this size for ten mornings. Every ten days, add a small amount of food to your previous breakfasts, until you've worked your way up to a normal-size breakfast. Be aware that for the first twenty days, due to the extremely small portion of food eaten, you will not be following our principles for firing up your metabolism by combining a grain carbohydrate with either a protein or a fat, unless you choose to eat a half serving of each. After twenty days of eating more food at breakfast, you then will never eat a grain carbohydrate without either a protein or a fat. Just be sure that after you have increased the size of your breakfast, it never contains more than one-third of your total daily food servings for the day. Remember, it is okay to eat fruit (carbohydrate) by itself if you plan to eat a larger meal in about an hour or two.

But Breakfast Makes Me Nauseous

Some of you may be saying, "I don't eat breakfast because my stomach can't handle food in the morning. The thought makes me nauseous." If this is you, first make sure that you are not feeling this way because you are taking vitamins, supplements, aspirin, birth-control pills, or any medication that should be eaten with food, on an empty stomach. Instead of increasing the amount of food you eat every ten days, as seen in the ten-day cycles for habitual breakfast banners starting on

> If you have been skipping breakfast, it is essential to change your habits *now* and start eating within one hour of awakening. If you continue to skip breakfast, you'll only make matters worse, slowing your metabolism more and more with every passing month.

page 142, try to eat something very small, such as half a banana or a slice of dry toast (don't have anything too acidic, such as an orange, as this may cause stomach discomfort), for one *entire* month, and do not skip even a day. You will grow accustomed to the small amount of food, and you'll be ready to get on track. Then start on the ten-day cycles.

Habitual Breakfast Banner's Ten-Day Cycle—Stage 1
CHOOSE ANY OPTION BELOW FOR TEN DAYS.

Bread
 Bread, whole wheat, $^1/_2$ slice
 Bread, whole wheat, reduced-calorie, 1 slice
 English muffin, $^1/_4$ muffin

Cereal (snack on dry cereal)
 All-Bran, extra fiber, $^1/_2$ cup
 All-Bran, original, $^1/_3$ cup
 Bran Flakes (Post), $^1/_3$ cup
 Cheerios, plain, $^1/_2$ cup
 Chex, Multi-Bran, $^1/_4$ cup
 Chex, Wheat, $^1/_3$ cup
 Fiber One, $^1/_2$ cup
 Frosted Mini-Wheats (Kellogg's), $1^1/_2$ biscuits
 Frosted Mini-Wheats Bite Size Cereal (Kellogg's), 6 biscuits
 Granola, low-fat, no sugar added, $^1/_8$ cup
 Grape-Nuts Flakes, $^1/_3$ cup
 Grape-Nuts, $^1/_8$ cup
 Kashi Go Lean, $^1/_3$ cup
 Kashi Good Friends, $^1/_2$ cup
 Kashi, Puffed, 7 whole grain and sesame, $^3/_4$ cups
 Life, $^1/_3$ cup
 Muesli, $^1/_6$ cup
 Nutri-Grain, corn, $^1/_3$ cup
 Nutri-Grain, wheat, $^1/_3$ cup
 Nutri-Grain Golden Wheat (Kellogg's), $^1/_3$ cup

Oat bran hot cereal, $^1/_4$ cup, cooked

Oatmeal, instant or slow-cooked oats, regular (Quaker), $^1/_4$ cup, cooked

Raisin Bran (Kellogg's and Post), $^1/_4$ cup

Raisin Bran (Total), $^1/_3$ cup

Ralston 100% Wheat Hot Cereal, $^1/_4$ cup, cooked

Roman Meal, $^1/_4$ cup, cooked

Shredded Wheat (Post), $^1/_3$ cup

Shredded Wheat N' Bran (Post), $^1/_3$ cup

Total, $^1/_3$ cup

Wheatena, $^1/_4$ cup, cooked

Wheaties, $^1/_2$ cup

Wheaties, Energy Crunch, $^1/_4$ cup

Fruit

Apple, $^1/_2$ medium

Banana, $^1/_2$ medium

Berries, $^1/_4$ cup

Chopped, cooked, or canned, $^1/_2$ cup

Dried, $^1/_8$ cup

Melon, small wedge

Yogurt

Nonfat, plain, $^1/_2$ cup

Nonfat, sugar-free, $^1/_2$ cup

Habitual Breakfast Banner's Ten-Day Cycle—Stage 2

CHOOSE ANY OPTION BELOW FOR TEN DAYS.

Bread (dry or with I Can't Believe It's Not Butter spray)

Bread, whole wheat, 1 slice

Bread, whole wheat, reduced calorie, 2 slices

English muffin, $^1/_2$ muffin

Cereal

All-Bran, extra fiber, 1 cup

All-Bran, original, $^3/_4$ cup

Bran Flakes (Post), $^3/_4$ cup

Cheerios, plain, 1 cup

Chex, Multi-Bran, 1/2 cup

Chex, Wheat, 2/3 cup

Fiber One, 1 cup

Frosted Mini-Wheats (Kellogg's), 3 biscuits

Frosted Mini-Wheats Bite Size Cereal (Kellogg's), 12 biscuits

Granola, low-fat, no sugar added, 1/4 cup

Grape Nut Flakes, 3/4 cup

Grape-Nuts, 1/4 cup

Kashi Go Lean, 3/4 cup

Kashi Good Friends, 1 cup

Kashi, Puffed, 7 whole grain and sesame, 1 1/3 cups

Life, 3/4 cup

Muesli, 1/3 cup

Nutri-Grain, corn, 2/3 cup

Nutri-Grain, wheat, 2/3 cup

Nutri-Grain Golden Wheat (Kellogg's), 3/4 cup

Oat bran hot cereal, 1/2 cup, cooked

Oatmeal, instant or slow-cooked oats, regular (Quaker), 1/2 cup, cooked

Raisin Bran (Kellogg's and Post), 1/2 cup

Raisin Bran (Total), 2/3 cup

Ralston 100% Wheat Hot Cereal, 1/2 cup, cooked

Roman Meal, 1/2 cup, cooked

Shredded Wheat (Post), 2/3 cup or 1 1/2 large biscuits

Shredded Wheat N' Bran (Post), 2/3 cup

Total, 3/4 cup

Wheatena, 1/2 cup, cooked

Wheaties, 1 cup

Wheaties, Energy Crunch, 1/2 cup

Fruit

Berries, 1/2 cup

Chopped, cooked, or canned, 1/2 cup

Dried, 1/4 cup

Melon, 1 wedge

Whole, such as a medium apple or small banana

Yogurt
  Low-fat, fruit added, with low-calorie sweetener, $1/2$ cup
  Nonfat, plain, 1 cup
  Nonfat, sugar-free, fruit-flavored, 1 cup

Habitual Breakfast Banner's Ten-Day Cycle—Stage 3

CHOOSE ANY OPTION FROM LIST A
("ALWAYS" CARBOHYDRATES) AND ANY OPTION FROM LIST B
("THUMBS-UP" PROTEINS OR "FRIENDLY" FATS) FOR TEN DAYS.

LIST A

Carbohydrates
  Bread (dry or with I Can't Believe It's Not Butter spray)
    Bread, whole wheat, 1 slice
    Bread, whole wheat, reduced-calorie, 2 slices
    English muffin, $1/2$ muffin

Cereal
    All-Bran, extra fiber, 1 cup
    All-Bran, original, $3/4$ cup
    Bran Flakes (Post), $3/4$ cup
    Cheerios, plain, 1 cup
    Chex, Multi-Bran, $1/2$ cup
    Chex, Wheat, $2/3$ cup
    Fiber One, 1 cup
    Frosted Mini-Wheats (Kellogg's), 3 biscuits
    Frosted Mini-Wheats Bite Size Cereal (Kellogg's), 12 biscuits
    Granola, low fat, no sugar added, $1/4$ cup
    Grape-Nuts Flakes, $3/4$ cup
    Grape-Nuts, $1/4$ cup
    Kashi Go Lean, $3/4$ cup
    Kashi Good Friends, 1 cup
    Kashi, Puffed, 7 whole grain and sesame, $1 1/3$ cups
    Life, $3/4$ cup

Muesli, $^1/_3$ cup

Nutri-Grain, corn, $^2/_3$ cup

Nutri-Grain, wheat, $^2/_3$ cup

Nutri-Grain Golden Wheat (Kellogg's), $^3/_4$ cup

Oat bran hot cereal, $^1/_2$ cup, cooked

Oatmeal, instant or slow-cooked oats, regular (Quaker), $^1/_2$ cup, cooked

Raisin Bran (Kellogg's and Post), $^1/_2$ cup

Raisin Bran (Total), $^2/_3$ cup

Ralston 100% Wheat Hot Cereal, $^1/_2$ cup, cooked

Roman Meal, $^1/_2$ cup, cooked

Shredded Wheat (Post), $^2/_3$ cup or $1^1/_2$ large biscuits

Shredded Wheat N' Bran (Post), $^2/_3$ cup

Total, $^3/_4$ cup

Wheatena, $^1/_2$ cup, cooked

Wheaties, 1 cup

Wheaties, Energy Crunch, $^1/_2$ cup

Fruit

Berries, $^1/_2$ cup

Chopped, cooked, or canned, $^1/_2$ cup

Dried fruit, $^1/_4$ cup

Melon, 1 wedge

Whole, such as medium apple or small banana

LIST B

Proteins

Bacon, Canadian, 1 long slice or 1 thin, round patty

Bacon, Canadian, extra lean, $1^1/_2$ long slices or $1^1/_2$ thin, round patties

Bacon, turkey, 1 long slice

Bacon, turkey, extra lean, $1^1/_2$ long slices

Cheese, low-fat and part-skim, all varieties, $^1/_3$ ounce

Cheese, nonfat and soy, all varieties, $^1/_2$ ounce

Cottage cheese, 1% fat and nonfat, $^1/_4$ cup

Egg, hard-boiled, $^1/_2$

Egg whites, 2

Milk, nonfat, 1%, and soy, $\frac{1}{3}$ cup
Yogurt, low-fat, fruit added, with low-calorie sweetener, $\frac{1}{4}$ cup
Yogurt, plain, nonfat, and sugar-free, $\frac{1}{2}$ cup

Fats

Fruits

Avocado, mashed, $\frac{1}{8}$ cup

Nuts

Almond butter, $1\frac{1}{2}$ flat teaspoons
Almonds, whole, 7
Brazil nuts, unblanched, 2
Cashew butter, 2 flat teaspoons
Cashews, dry or oil roasted, 6
Chestnuts, European, roasted, $\frac{1}{8}$ cup
Filberts/Hazelnuts, 6
Macadamias, roasted or dry roasted, 3
Mixed nuts, dry or oil roasted, 1 tablespoon
Peanut butter, $\frac{1}{2}$ flat tablespoon
Peanut butter, reduced fat, $\frac{1}{2}$ flat tablespoon
Peanuts, dry or oil roasted, 10 nuts or 1 tablespoon
Pecans, dry or oil roasted, 3 halves or 1 tablespoon
Pine nuts, dried, 1 tablespoon
Pistachios, dry roasted, $1\frac{3}{4}$ tablespoons
Pumpkin kernels, dried, 1 tablespoon
Sesame seeds, 1 tablespoon
Sunflower seeds, dry or oil roasted, 1 tablespoon
Tahini (sesame butter), $\frac{1}{2}$ flat teaspoon
Walnuts, black, chopped, 1 tablespoon
Walnuts, English, chopped, 4 nuts or 1 tablespoon

Oil

Canola, 1 teaspoon
Corn, 1 teaspoon
Olive, 1 teaspoon
Peanut, 1 teaspoon
Safflower, 1 teaspoon
Soybean, 1 teaspoon

Soybean/cottonseed, 1 teaspoon

Sunflower, 1 teaspoon

Spreads

Hummus, 1 1/2 flat tablespoons

Habitual Breakfast Banner's Ten-Day Cycle—Stage 4

CHOOSE ANY OPTION FROM LIST A
("ALWAYS" CARBOHYDRATES) AND ANY OPTION FROM LIST B
("THUMBS-UP" PROTEINS OR "FRIENDLY" FATS) FOR TEN DAYS.

LIST A

Carbohydrates

Bread (dry or with I Can't Believe It's Not Butter spray)

Bread, whole wheat, 1 slice

Bread, whole wheat, reduced-calorie, 2 slices

English muffin, 1/2 muffin

Cereal

All-Bran, extra fiber, 1 cup

All-Bran, original, 3/4 cup

Bran Flakes (Post), 3/4 cup

Cheerios, plain, 1 cup

Chex, Multi-Bran, 1/2 cup

Chex, Wheat, 2/3 cup

Fiber One, 1 cup

Frosted Mini-Wheats (Kellogg's), 3 biscuits

Frosted Mini-Wheats Bite Size Cereal (Kellogg's), 12 biscuits

Granola, low-fat, no sugar added, 1/4 cup

Grape-Nuts Flakes, 3/4 cup

Grape-Nuts, 1/4 cup

Kashi Go Lean, 3/4 cup

Kashi Good Friends, 1 cup

Kashi, Puffed, 7 whole grain and sesame, 1 1/3 cups

Life, 3/4 cup

Muesli, 1/3 cup

Nutri-Grain, corn, $^2/_3$ cup

Nutri-Grain, wheat, $^2/_3$ cup

Nutri-Grain Golden Wheat (Kellogg's), $^3/_4$ cup

Oat bran hot cereal, $^1/_2$ cup, cooked

Oatmeal, instant or slow-cooked oats, regular (Quaker), $^1/_2$ cup, cooked

Raisin Bran (Kellogg's and Post), $^1/_2$ cup

Raisin Bran (Total), $^2/_3$ cup

Ralston 100% Wheat Hot Cereal, $^1/_2$ cup, cooked

Roman Meal, $^1/_2$ cup, cooked

Shredded Wheat (Post), $^2/_3$ cup or $1^1/_2$ large biscuits

Shredded Wheat N' Bran (Post), $^2/_3$ cup

Total, $^3/_4$ cup

Wheatena, $^1/_2$ cup, cooked

Wheaties, 1 cup

Wheaties, Energy Crunch, $^1/_2$ cup

Fruit

Berries, $^1/_2$ cup

Chopped, cooked, or canned, $^1/_2$ cup

Dried, $^1/_4$ cup

Melon, 1 wedge

Whole, such as medium apple or small banana

LIST B

Proteins

Bacon, Canadian, 2 long slices or 2 thin, round patties

Bacon, Canadian, extra lean, 3 long slices or 3 thin, round patties

Bacon, turkey, 2 long slices

Bacon, turkey, extra lean, 3 long slices

Cheese, low-fat and part-skim, all varieties, $^3/_4$ ounce

Cheese, nonfat and soy, all varieties, 1 ounce

Cottage cheese, 1% fat and nonfat, $^1/_2$ cup

Egg, hard-boiled, 1

Egg whites, 4

Milk, nonfat, 1%, and soy, $^3/_4$ cup

Yogurt, plain, nonfat, and sugar-free, 1 cup

Yogurt, low-fat, fruit added, with low-calorie sweetener, $^1/_2$ cup

Fats

Fruits
Avocado, mashed, 1/4 cup

Nuts
Almond butter, 1 flat tablespoon
Almonds, whole, 14
Brazil nuts, unblanched, 4
Cashew butter, 1 flat tablespoon
Cashews, dry or oil roasted, 11
Chestnuts, European, roasted, 1/4 cup
Filberts/hazelnuts, 11
Macadamias, roasted or dry roasted, 5 nuts or 1/2 tablespoon
Mixed nuts, dry or oil roasted, 2 tablespoons
Peanut butter, 1 flat tablespoon
Peanut butter, reduced fat, 1 flat tablespoon
Peanuts, dry or oil roasted, 20 nuts or 2 tablespoons
Pecans, dry or oil roasted, 7 halves or 2 tablespoons
Pine nuts, dried, 2 tablespoons
Pistachios, dry roasted, 2 1/2 tablespoons
Pumpkin kernels, dried, 2 tablespoons
Sesame seeds, 2 tablespoons
Sunflower seeds, dry or oil roasted, 2 tablespoons
Tahini (sesame butter), 1 flat tablespoon
Walnuts, black, chopped, 2 tablespoons
Walnuts, English, chopped, 8 nuts or 2 tablespoons

Oils
Canola, 2 teaspoons
Corn, 2 teaspoons
Olive, 2 teaspoons
Peanut, 2 teaspoons
Safflower, 2 teaspoons
Soybean, 2 teaspoons
Soybean/cottonseed, 2 teaspoons
Sunflower, 2 teaspoons

Spreads
Hummus, 3 flat tablespoons

Once you start to eat breakfast, you may experience hunger later in the morning. Believe it or not, this is actually great news! It means that your metabolism has sped up and your body is burning fat and calories more efficiently. You may want to start having a slightly larger breakfast or start eating a small midmorning snack. You may need to eat a little less at another meal, but just make sure that at the end of the day, you have not consumed more than your total daily servings of carbohydrates, proteins, and fats.

SEVEN

Missing Meals: Misdemeanor or Manslaughter?

Myth Busters

MYTH: People who skip meals eat less than other people and they will always be lean.

BUSTED: People who skip meals binge and overeat at their next meal, often consuming more calories than they would have consumed if they hadn't skipped a meal. Also, when you skip meals your body goes into a semi-starvation mode. In an attempt to conserve fuel, the metabolism slows and fat and calories are burned at a very slow rate. This makes a fat body, not a lean one.

MYTH: If you haven't eaten in a long time, it's good if you don't feel hungry.

BUSTED: This is bad. It is a true sign that your metabolism has slowed. By making it a habit to wait a long time to eat, your body adjusts; it expects to wait to be fed and therefore conserves fuel by burning very few calories. When you haven't eaten and your body no longer senses hunger, it means your metabolism has slowed.

MYTH: If you get home late, it's best to go to bed without eating dinner.

BUSTED: Although a late dinner should be small and light, you need to keep your metabolism revved by eating. This prevents your body from feeling threatened and as though it may starve to death.

In college, our friends used to boast about their eating habits. "I skipped lunch, and now I'm going to treat myself and have a huge dinner!" Or, "I've been so good today. All I've eaten is a piece of fruit, so now I can have as much as I want tonight when we go out to the Cheesecake Factory." We suspected that our friends were misguided and that their diet plans were backfiring.

After witnessing clients who had the same habits as our college friends and helping them to fire up their metabolism by eating regularly, we were certain that skipping meals really does slow the burning of calories and contribute to an increase in body fat. To see how much we would be affected, we conducted our twin trial.

Our Twin Trial
in which you see that the more often you eat, the more pounds you lose

Tammy: I lost the flip. I was to be the guinea pig for six weeks as we tested the theory that eating only two or three large meals during the day would affect my metabolism, causing me to store body fat and gain weight more readily than if I were eating my usual five to six small meals/snacks throughout the day.

I changed my habits so that I ate the same amount of food but in only three meals. My usual minimeals/snacks of yogurt, bell pepper strips with hummus, or whole wheat crackers with nonfat cheese were added to the main meals. My exercise regimen and other daily habits remained the same.

I immediately noticed that my energy levels dipped in the midafternoon. I also was constantly hungry. By lunch and by dinner I was ravenous, which caused me to eat very quickly. Then, when I was finished with my meals, I never felt satisfied, even though the meals themselves were larger than I was accustomed to. I wanted to eat more, but that would jeopardize the results of the trial. To make matters worse, I experienced other negative side effects.

I was irritable. There are minor things New Yorkers grow accustomed to and don't allow to bother them. The squeaking of subway wheels, the tourists who walk leisurely on the streets enjoying the sights as you rush to get past them, the occasional city smell—these are all things that become part of New Yorkers' everyday lives. Well, suddenly, all of these minor things were a major deal, and I didn't hesitate to speak my mind. The squeaking subway seemed more like the constant sound of fingernails scratching on a blackboard. The leisurely tourists seemed more like obstacle courses that were always in my way. In fact, one day I was tempted to push a man who was simply standing directly in my path. The occasional city smell was magnified to the point where I grunted and made horrible faces.

I also experienced cravings. This added to my irritability, as I wasn't allowed to give in to them. The cravings were weirdly specific: a lemon poppy-seed muffin, a black and white cookie, or an Almond Joy candy bar (a Mounds absolutely wouldn't do). I attributed my cravings to my seemingly insatiable hunger. To try to break the intensity of my cravings, I drank Crystal Light or diet soda in order to get a little bit of sweet flavor without the calories of the treats I actually craved. The drinks didn't help much—I remained cranky.

At the end of the six weeks, my body fat had increased 2 percent and I had gained 1.9 pounds. This is amazing, given that I had eaten the same exact amount of food as usual, just not spread throughout the day. And my exercise regime hadn't changed. Even though we had expected to see negative results, we were surprised to see such a change after only six weeks.

Reaping the Benefits of Eating Frequently

Many people who bulk their day's food into three (or even two) large meals have come to us seeking help. Cathy, a forty-eight-year-old woman, claimed that she had always struggled with her weight. At twenty, she became a flight attendant. At that time, regardless of height, her airline required flight attendants to weigh fewer than 125 pounds. At five foot five, it was a constant battle for Cathy to try to achieve that weight. For weeks before the weigh-ins, Cathy ate just celery sticks, carrots, and diet soda. The rest of the year, she tried to eat just once or twice a day, only to feel humiliated at weigh-ins when she was usually above the rigid standards. Moreover, each year, Cathy's weight was higher and her clothes were tighter, and attaining that 125-pound goal ultimately became impossible. By the time she came to us, the airlines had abandoned these weight requirements, and Cathy no longer lived on rabbit food; however, she still ate only one or two meals a day and felt almost constantly deprived, yet she was heavier than ever. We instantly put Cathy on our Fire Up Your Metabolism plan, in which she would eat five to six small meals. At our initial session, Cathy was afraid that eating more meals would mean more body fat and more weight. But Cathy was ecstatic when, to her amazement, she had lost seventeen pounds and was a lean 128 pounds after just two months. After following our plan, Cathy said that she "could eat like a human being" and was finally losing weight without a struggle as she had sped up her metabolism.

TIP

WHOA, NELLY! IS THAT YOUR MIDMORNING GRUMBLING BELLY? SAY GOOD-BYE TO TOAST AND JELLY. You need a midmorning snack that keeps hunger at bay and has a metabolism-revving combination of energy-boosting carbohydrates with satiating protein or fat. Choose any of the following snacks and you will surely fire it up!

- ¾ cup Kashi Go Lean cereal and ¾ cup skim milk or soy milk

- ½ whole wheat pita stuffed with ½ cup 1 percent fat or nonfat cottage cheese, sprinkled with a dash of cinnamon

- 1 cup nonfat, sugar-free yogurt (or ½ cup nonfat, sugar-added or low-fat yogurt) with ¼ cup Grape-Nuts sprinkled on top

- One 4-inch whole wheat Aunt Jemima waffle and 1 flat tablespoon peanut butter or soy butter

- ½ cup oatmeal and ¾ cup skim milk or soy milk

- 2 cups of Health Valley Organic Lentil, Italian Minestrone, or Lentil and Carrot soup; or 1¾ cups of Health Valley Split Pea or Split Pea and Carrots; or 1½ cups of Black Bean and Vegetable

- One scrambled egg on one slice of whole wheat toast or on half a whole wheat English muffin (no butter or oil on pan for egg!)

- ½ cup cubed cantaloupe with ½ cup nonfat or low-fat cottage cheese, sprinkled with cinnamon

- Carrot sticks and 2 tablespoons hummus or low-fat string cheese

- Line a celery stalk with 1 flat tablespoon peanut butter or soy butter and add 2 tablespoons raisins

- Half a whole wheat English muffin and 1 ounce low-fat cheese

Eat More Frequently, Weigh Less

As ironic as it sounds, when you eat more frequently, you burn more calories. The key to firing up your metabolism is to eat more often than you were, but not more food than you were (at least not yet).

WHEN IT COMES TO CHIPS, SEAL THOSE LIPS! Most chips get the majority of their calories from fat. If you filled up on these low-fiber, calorie-dense snacks, by the time you finally felt satiated, you would have gotten a whopping amount of calories and over-whelmed your metabolism. (Soy chips are an exception to the chip rule, as calories come from protein and carbs and most of the chips even contain fiber. Banana chips, however, are fried.)

SMASH THAT SMOOTHIE FOR A SNACK HABIT. Some smoothies pack in as many as thirteen hundred calories—almost as many calories as some people need for the entire day!

LOVE FETA CHEESE? You can make feta a healthy option! Stuff $3/4$ ounce low-fat feta cheese, sprouts, tomato, and lettuce in half a whole wheat pita.

JUST POP IT AND TOP IT. Top 3 cups air-popped popcorn with cinnamon, I Can't Believe It's Not Butter *spray*, Butter Buds, or Mrs. Dash, and 1 tablespoon soy nuts, walnuts, or pecans.

DID SOMEBODY SAY CHEESY TOMATO SOUP? Make your own healthy version by melting 1 ounce nonfat cheese in $1^{1}/_{2}$ cups Health Valley Tomato soup.

THIS 3:00 SNACK EVERY DAY WILL KEEP THE DOCTOR AWAY. Slice an apple and spread 1 flat tablespoon peanut butter on top. The apple gives you that energy-boosting, fiber-filled punch while the fat in the peanut butter helps keep you satiated for a little bit longer. Not to mention, peanuts are a great way to get some extra folic acid and fiber.

CHEESE AND CRACKERS CAN MAKE THE PERFECT SNACK. Just be sure they are either Health Valley Whole Wheat crackers, Finn

Crisps, or Hain's Wheatettes and eat just one serving (according to the box) with one ounce soy cheese or nonfat cheese.

JUST A PIECE OF FRUIT BETTER NOT BE YOUR AFTERNOON SNACK. When you follow our Fire Up Your Metabolism mini-meal tips you never overeat at one sitting. This means that when you eat your afternoon snack, you need more than just an apple unaccompanied by protein or fat to tide you over until dinnertime. (If you snack on just a piece of fruit, you'll be ravenous at dinner and will inevitably end up overeating.) However, there are two exceptions to this rule: 1) you had a larger lunch than you should have and you have just a few food servings left for the day, or 2) you plan to have another small snack (or dinner) within an hour or two after eating a piece of fruit. Just don't make the first exception a habit.

SOUP IT UP AN HOUR OR TWO BEFORE EATING DINNER OUT. Research shows that eating soup as a premeal significantly reduces the amount of calories you consume at the following meal. Choose low-calorie soups such as gazpacho, minestrone, and other vegetable-based soups.

A TASTE OF MEXICO. Mix $\frac{1}{2}$ cup brown rice and $\frac{1}{2}$ cup black beans. Well, in Mexico they may not use brown rice, but you should. This protein-carbohydrate combination is fiber-filled and will keep your energy high and your metabolism fired up.

EDAMAME BEANS ARE SURE TO KEEP YOU LEAN AND YOUNG LIKE YOU WERE IN YOUR TEENS. These fresh soybeans in a pod have a winning mixture of carbs and protein. They not only provide you with energy and a metabolic-boosting blast but also have about sixty calories and three grams of fiber per $\frac{1}{2}$ cup of pods. They will fill your stomach, keeping you satiated until dinnertime.

Put Off Eating, Slow Your Metabolism

When you wait too long to eat, your metabolism slows. You see, your body is very smart, and when you don't eat for a while, your body thinks you may starve to death. (This is the same as the metabolic slowing that occurs overnight.) Therefore, your body starts to conserve its fuel, burning fat and calories very slowly as a protective mechanism. When you do eat and finally give your body the fuel that it is looking for, it says, "Hey, I am not going to starve to death!" And once again it starts to freely burn fat and calories for energy, and diet-induced thermogenesis begins.

Eating Infrequently Overwhelms Your Metabolism, Even If You Don't Overeat

Most people who wait a long time to eat feel ravenous when they finally do eat, and they wind up eating much more food than they should. But even if you give your body a normal-size meal after waiting a very long time to eat, your body, as happy as it is to receive food, says, "Well, I'm glad I got fed, but I can't possibly handle this much food right now. After all, just moments before I was in a conservation mode, trying to hold on to whatever calories and fat I could. What am I supposed to do with all of this food now?" Your body winds up storing some of these calories as fat rather than burning them up for energy.

If you had eaten part of this meal a few hours earlier, the food would have been burned up for energy. The continuous food supply would have allowed the diet-induced thermogenesis to keep your metabolism fired up all day while also preventing your body from feeling the threat of starvation. In addition, you would have provided yourself with a consistent source of energy, avoiding mood swings and that uncomfortable belly grumbling. Also, you would have prevented yourself from becoming ravenous and thus not indulged in large portions of food at your next meal.

Research supports that eating small, frequent meals throughout the day is beneficial to a speedy metabolism and losing weight. Skipping meals leads to weight gain and a depressed metabolic rate. A study published in the *International Journal of Obesity and Related Metabolic Disorders* compared the impact of feeding adult men one-third of their daily calories between breakfast and dinner in one meal or in several small meals. For example, if lunch was normally three cups of spaghetti and meatballs, this was divided up so that one cup was eaten earlier than usual, one cup was eaten at the normal lunchtime, and one cup was eaten a couple of hours after the normal lunchtime. The results of this study confirm those of many similar studies—including our twin trial. The men whose lunchtime meal was divided into several small meals and eaten throughout the day consumed 27 percent fewer calories at dinner (which was given 5½ hours after the single meal) than those who ate the lunch as a single meal. Eating smaller, more frequent meals helps people to feel satisfied while consuming fewer calories, thereby leading to weight loss.

See the sidebar on pages 165 to 166 for some examples of how you can spread out your lunch so that you will eat less later.

Fueling for Exercise

Remember, carbohydrates are the fuel for your muscles. Therefore, you need to eat them before your workout (depending on the size of your meal, allow at least forty-five minutes to an hour for digestion). Also, be sure to follow the Fire Up Your Metabolism principles and include a little bit of protein or a little fat with your carbohydrate.

TIPS FOR PRE-EXERCISE SNACKS

DON'T EVEN THINK ABOUT THAT PROTEIN BAR AN HOUR BEFORE EXERCISE! Carbohydrates, not protein, provide your body with energy. You need to choose a pre-exercise snack that contains plenty of carbohydrates and some protein. (Actually, you shouldn't think about protein bars at all.)

THERE'S NOTHING BETTER THAN PEANUT BUTTER . . . EXCEPT ALMOND BUTTER OR CASHEW BUTTER! Spread 1 flat tablespoon of any nut butter on half a whole wheat English muffin for a snack that is sure to give you a jump-start.

TRAIL MIX FOR YOUR EVERYDAY LIFE. Place 4 apricots and 11 cashews in little plastic zipper bags so they are ready to go with you on your hectic days.

A DIFFERENT KIND OF TRAIL MIX: 1 cup Multi-Bran Chex or Cheerios and 14 almonds or 7 pecan halves.

YOUR NEW TRAVELING COMPANION TASTES GREAT AND TRAVELS WELL. Prepackage 2 large tablespoons raisins with 2 tablespoons peanuts, sunflower seeds, or pistachios.

MAKE AN OPEN-FACED BURGER. Try one veggie Boca Burger or Gardenburger on half a whole wheat bun. Top with lettuce, tomato, onions, any other veggies you like, and a little bit of ketchup.

AS LONG AS THERE'S NO COUCH, IT'S GOOD IN OUR BOOK. The potato, that is. A great pre-exercise snack is a three-ounce baked potato topped with 1/2 cup nonfat or low-fat cottage cheese and broccoli. (If your body doesn't handle dairy well before exercise, you may want to try one of the other snacks.)

A Shrinking Stomach—a Growing Case for Small, Frequent Meals

Eating small, frequent meals has benefits. Have you ever tried a diet in which you ate much smaller portions than usual? After a couple of weeks, you probably started to feel full much sooner than you did before you started the diet. This feeling of fullness is another advantage to eating smaller, more frequent meals—your stomach capacity is likely to shrink. A study that examined the stomach capacity of people on a diet (eating smaller portions at each sitting) for four weeks showed that stomach capacity was reduced by 27 to 36 percent compared to control subjects who maintained their usual eating habits. This suggests that people who regularly eat smaller, more frequent meals begin to feel more satisfied eating smaller portions at a meal.

In addition, reducing your caloric intake by 10 percent a day, while adding an extra meal, revs your metabolism and causes you to lose as much as five pounds per month.

TIPS FOR AFTER-DINNER SNACKS

WHAT'S THE BEST TIME FOR EIGHT OUNCES OF WARM SKIM MILK? When you are hungry two hours before bed. Mom was right. This drink helps to put you to sleep, as it is rich in calcium and therefore helps to soothe you by causing your muscles to relax.

BRIDGE MIX IS A BETTER SNACK THAN GUMMY BEARS. Gummy bears will give you a sugar high followed by a sugar crash, along with intense cravings for more simple and refined carbohydrates. The nuts in bridge mix contain protein and fat, which slows digestion, keeping you satiated longer and helping to provide a steady source of energy. Both snacks, however, are far from ideal.

Staying on Track with Your Snacks

The importance of eating several small meals and snacks throughout the day is clear. However, the timing of these snacks, and the foods you choose for them is *critical*.

Before we begin to discuss the times at which these snacks must be eaten, we need to clarify what we mean by "snack." We prefer to call these snacks "minimeals," because "snack" has lousy connotations. When it comes to eating a mini-meal, we do not mean that you should sit down to a bag of potato chips or grab a brownie. There are specific foods that provide your body with a powerful, metabolic-boosting punch. That said, we use the words "snacks" and "mini-meals" interchangeably in hopes of your relearning what constitutes a snack.

PERFORM PORTION CONTROL CHECKUPS. Once a week, measure out the portions you are eating to make sure that you aren't getting more than you should.

NEVER DO IT HUNGRY—GROCERY SHOP, THAT IS. When you're hungry, it is nearly impossible to turn down unhealthy temptations and you wind up stocking your shelves with excess "rarely" carbohydrates, "thumbs-down" proteins, and fat "foes."

PUT DOWN YOUR FORK BETWEEN BITES. It will slow you down. It takes twenty minutes for your brain to receive the signal that your stomach is full. A lot of damage and excess calories can be consumed in that time.

STUFFED AND ROASTED? THAT'S YOU IF YOU ALLOW YOURSELF TO FEEL EXTREMELY FULL AFTER EVERY MEAL. Avoid getting to the point where you are so full that your waistband feels tight. Allow your stomach to shrink and you will feel satiated more easily.

USE SMALLER PLATES. Most people make a habit of filling their plates. Bigger plates mean bigger meals and bigger bellies.

LOAD UP ON A VEGGIE PREMEAL. Fill up on nutrient- and fiber-packed, low-calorie vegetables and you will eat less at the following meal.

STOP AND RELAX. For two to three minutes in the middle of your meal, stop. It will make you aware of how full you actually are, and you may reevaluate and realize that you don't need more food.

FEED THE HUNGRY. Clear your refrigerator and pantry of high-calorie and fatty snacks. If they are unopened, donate them to a local shelter or food bank. If they are opened, throw them away. Out of sight, out of mind.

Fire Up Your Metabolism by Appropriately Timing Your Snacks

Time your snacks so that you are never waiting longer than four to five hours to eat. You should aim to have a mini-meal every two to four hours. This provides a constant source of fuel for your body so that it never feels threatened into conserving calories and fat. When you consistently give your body food, diet-induced thermogenesis constantly occurs and you are burning calories throughout the entire day. What's more, you never feel ravenous and, therefore, you don't binge. Finally, a continuous supply of energy prevents peaks and valleys in energy levels as well as mood swings. This allows you to have more energy for everyday activities as well as for exercise.

Plan your day so that you never wait more than five hours between meals/snacks. If you know that you have a busy day and will be eating a late dinner, eat your afternoon snack later in the day. For example, if you usually eat lunch at noon, your afternoon snack at 3:00 P.M. and dinner at 6:00, but today, you won't be able to eat dinner until 8:30, make sure to schedule your midafternoon snack for 4:00 or 4:30.

Adding Extra Meals: Isn't Weight Gain Inevitable?

The key to burning extra calories all day long is to spread out the *same amount of food* (calories) that you normally eat. Do not make the mistake of eating more food than you were before. If you simply

Eating at a restaurant? Before you even receive your meal, ask that half of it be doggie-bagged for you to take home. Portion sizes are usually very large, and they add too much fat and too many calories into your day, throwing your metabolism into overdrive. Save half of your meal for the next day.

added snacks into your normal routine, you would be increasing your daily calories, and this would backfire. You won't be eating a full meal every four hours. Smaller, well-balanced mini-meals are the goal.

For example, if you usually eat a turkey sandwich, a banana, and a low-fat yogurt at lunch, split it into three parts. Eat either the yogurt or half of the turkey sandwich for a midmorning snack, save one-third for your lunch, and save one-third for your midafternoon snack. (Just be sure to follow our guidelines for mixing the right amounts of the best carbohydrates, proteins, and fats.) Or, you could eat half of your normal lunch, then choose your morning and afternoon snacks from our Snack Lists (see the table on pages 168–176). Both options are great—you eat the same amount of food as before, yet you burn more calories.

How can you spread out your lunch so that you burn more calories and also eat less later? It's easy. Here are examples of typical lunchtime meals and ways to spread them out, enhancing your efforts to fire up your metabolism.

Typical lunchtime meal: Grilled chicken sandwich, side salad of greens with nonfat dressing, orange
Spread it out: One and a half hours before lunch, eat half of the salad and half of the orange. At lunchtime, eat half of the sandwich and the other half of the orange. About three to four hours later, eat the other half of the sandwich and the other half of the salad.

Typical lunchtime meal: Lentil soup, baked potato with a dollop of nonfat yogurt and chives, and a side of steamed veggies

Spread it out: Eat half of the lentil soup with half of the steamed veggies two hours before normal lunchtime, have the other half of the soup and half of the yogurt-topped potato at lunchtime, and have the remaining yogurt-topped potato and veggies three to four hours later.

Typical lunchtime meal: Pasta with grilled shrimp and calamari, loaded with tons of broccoli (entire meal is three cups); a side of carrot, zucchini, bell pepper, cucumber, and celery strips (also totaling three cups)

Spread it out: Divide pasta and veggies into three equal portions. Have one portion two hours before lunch, one portion at lunchtime, and the last portion three to four hours later.

Hindering Habits

Identify your habit that is preventing you from keeping your metabolism as speedy as it should be. After you locate your "hindering habit," follow the guidelines below your current habit to meet the specific needs of your depressed metabolism.

You eat only three times per day (breakfast, lunch, dinner). Choose either option 1 or 2 below. Whichever option you choose, you must stick to it for the entire day.

	Midmorning	Lunch	Midafternoon	Dinner
Option 1	Eat ¹/₃ of your usual lunch.	Eat ¹/₃ of your usual lunch.	Eat ¹/₃ of your usual lunch.	No changes necessary but see previous chapters for which food you should choose.

Option 2	Choose one of our snacks from snack lists on pages 168 to 176.	Eat ½ of your usual lunch (save other ½ for tomorrow).	Choose one of our snacks from snack lists on pages 168 to 176.	No changes necessary but see previous chapters for which foods you should choose.

You eat only two times per day (lunch and dinner). Choose either option 1 or 2 below. Whichever option you choose, you must stick to it for the entire day.

	Morning	Lunch	Midafternoon	Dinner
Option 1	Eat ½ of your lunch.	Eat remaining ½ of your lunch.	Choose one of our snacks. (Ideally, you'd eat ½ of dinner now, but this is not feasible if you work outside the home.)	Eat ½ of your usual dinner.
Option 2	Choose one of our snacks.	Eat ½ of your usual lunch or one of our snacks.	Choose one of our snacks. (Ideally, you'd eat ½ of dinner now, but this is not feasible if you work outside the home.)	Eat ½ of your usual dinner.

You eat three meals a day and only one snack. Choose either option 1 or 2. Whichever option you choose, you must stick to it for the entire day.

	Morning	Lunch	Midafternoon	Dinner
Option 1	Choose one of our snacks.	Eat your usual lunch.	Choose one of our snacks.	Eat ⅔ of your usual dinner.
Option 2	Choose one of our snacks.	Eat ⅔ of your usual lunch.	Choose one of our snacks.	Eat your usual dinner.

You eat three meals a day and one or more high-calorie snacks (such as a candy bar, doughnut, pastry, cookies, or 200 calories or more of chips). Follow the guidelines below.

Midmorning	Lunch	Midafternoon	Dinner
Choose one of our snacks.	Eat $^3/_4$ of your usual lunch.	Choose one of our snacks.	Eat $^3/_4$ of your usual dinner.

You skip two meals out of three (you usually eat just lunch or just dinner; you probably drink a lot of coffee or soda during the day, too, to give you the energy you're not getting from food). Follow the guidelines below.

Midmorning	Lunch	Midafternoon	Dinner
Choose one of our snacks.	Choose one of our snacks.	Choose one of our snacks.	Choose one of our snacks.

Snack/Mini-Meal Lists

For protein serving sizes, see pages 33 to 35 to find out what part of the hand each serving size is equivalent to.

Note: These snack portions are for people on the lowest levels of the Fire Up Your Metabolism plan. Your snacks can be bigger; just be sure that at the end of the day you don't exceed your daily food servings.

CHOOSE ANY ONE OPTION FROM LIST A
AND ANY ONE OPTION FROM LIST B.

LIST A

Carbohydrates

Breads

Bread, pumpernickel (label must say "whole" pumpernickel), 1 slice

Bread, whole-grain rye, 1 slice

Bread, whole wheat, 1 slice

English muffin, oat bran, $^1/_2$ muffin

English muffin, whole wheat, $1/2$ muffin

Matzo, Manischewitz 100% whole wheat, 1 piece

Pita, whole wheat, $1/2$ of large pita

Tortilla, whole wheat, 6–8" diameter, 1

Breakfast Grains: Pancakes and Waffles

Pancakes, whole wheat, 4" diameter, 1

Pancakes, whole wheat, Arrowhead Mills, 4" diameter, 1

Pancakes, whole wheat, Aunt Jemima (although not entirely whole wheat, it is more whole wheat than white flour), 4" diameter, 1

Waffles, Eggo Nutri-Grain Multigrain, 1

Waffles, Van's 7 Grain Whole Wheat (one of the few times when seven-grain is 100% whole grain!), 1

Cereals: Make your own trail mix by mixing a cereal serving with nuts from List B. Prebag your snack and bring wherever you go.

All-Bran, extra fiber, 1 cup

All-Bran, original, $3/4$ cup

Bran Flakes (Post), $3/4$ cup

Cheerios, plain, 1 cup

Chex, Multi-Bran, $1/2$ cup

Chex, Wheat, $2/3$ cup

Fiber One, 1 cup

Frosted Mini-Wheats (Kellogg's), 3 biscuits

Frosted Mini-Wheats Bite Size Cereal (Kellogg's), 12 biscuits

Granola, low fat, no sugar added, $1/4$ cup

Grape-Nuts Flakes, $3/4$ cup

Grape-Nuts, $1/4$ cup

Honey Frosted Mini-Wheats, 12 biscuits

Kashi Go Lean, $3/4$ cup

Kashi Good Friends, 1 cup

Kashi, Puffed, 7 whole grain and sesame, $1 1/3$ cups

Life, $3/4$ cup

Muesli, $1/3$ cup

Nutri-Grain, corn, $2/3$ cup

Nutri-Grain, wheat, $2/3$ cup

Nutri-Grain Golden Wheat (Kellogg's), $3/4$ cup

Oat bran hot cereal, $1/2$ cup, cooked

Oatmeal, instant or slow-cooked oats, regular (Quaker), $^1/_2$ cup, cooked

Raisin Bran (Kellogg's and Post), $^1/_2$ cup

Raisin Bran (Total), $^2/_3$ cup

Ralston 100% Wheat Hot Cereal, $^1/_2$ cup, cooked

Roman Meal, $^1/_2$ cup, cooked

Shredded Wheat (Post), $^2/_3$ cup or $1^1/_2$ large biscuits

Shredded Wheat N' Bran (Post), $^2/_3$ cup

Total, $^3/_4$ cup

Wheatena, $^1/_2$ cup, cooked

Wheaties, 1 cup

Wheaties, Energy Crunch, $^1/_2$ cup

Crackers

Ak-Mak, 5 slices

Ry Krisp, 3 items

Rye wafers, whole grain, 3 crackers

Wasa Organic Rye Original Crispbread, 4 slices

Wasa Original Whole Wheat Crispbread, 2 slices

Whole wheat (Health Valley), 10 crackers

Whole wheat wafers, 4 wafers

Fruits

Apple, 1 small

Applesauce, unsweetened, $^1/_2$ cup

Apricots, 4

Bananas, 1 small or $^1/_2$ large

Blackberries, $^1/_2$ cup

Blueberries, $^1/_2$ cup

Canned fruit, $^1/_2$ cup

Cantaloupe, $^1/_2$ whole

Cherries, $^3/_4$ cup

Dried fruit, $^1/_4$ cup

Grapefruit, $^1/_2$ large or 1 small

Grapes, 20

Honeydew, 1 wedge ($^1/_8$ of melon)

Kiwi, $1^1/_2$

Mango, ½ large

Nectarine, 1 large

Orange, 1 large

Peach, 1 large

Pear, 1 small

Pineapple chunks, ½ cup

Strawberries, ½ cup sliced or 1 cup whole

Grains (cooked)

Barley, ½ cup

Buckwheat groats (kasha), ½ cup

Bulgur, whole grain, ½ cup

Pasta, whole wheat, ½ cup

Quinoa, ½ cup

Rice, brown, ½ cup

Popcorn and Pretzels

Popcorn, air-popped, 3 cups

Popcorn, Bearitos, no salt, no oil, 4 cups popped

Popcorn, Healthy Choice, 6 cups popped

Pretzels, whole wheat, 1 large, equal to 80–100 calories

Soup

Garden Vegetables, Health Valley, 2 cups

Minestrone, Health Valley, 1½ cups

Mushroom Barley, Health Valley, 1½ cups

Potato Leek, Health Valley, 1½ cups

Tomato, Health Valley, 1½ cups

Vegetable Barley, Health Valley, 1½ cups

Vegetables: All vegetables can be eaten in unlimited amounts (as long as sauce is not added; for example, do not add dressings, butter, oils, etc.), with the exception of peas, potatoes, and corn.

Corn, 1 medium ear

Peas, ½ cup

Potato, baked, 3 ounces

Proteins

Beans

Beans, all varieties, $^1/_2$ cup

Edamame, with shells, $^2/_3$ cup

Dairy

Cheese, low-fat, all varieties, $^3/_4$ ounce (1 prepackaged slice)

Cheese, nonfat, all varieties, 1 ounce

Cottage cheese, 2% fat, $^1/_4$ cup

Cottage cheese, 1% fat or nonfat, $^1/_2$ cup

Egg, hard-boiled, 1

Egg whites, 4

Feta, low-fat, $^3/_4$ ounce

Milk, 1% and nonfat, $^3/_4$ cup

Mozzarella, nonfat, 1 ounce

Mozzarella, part skim, $^3/_4$ ounce (1 prepackaged slice)

Soy cheese, nonfat, 1 ounce

Soy cheese, full-fat, $^3/_4$ ounce

Soy milk, full-fat and low-fat, $^3/_4$ cup

String cheese, low-fat, $1^1/_2$ items

Yogurt, full-fat, $^1/_3$ cup

Yogurt, low-fat, $^1/_2$ cup

Yogurt, nonfat, sugar added, $^3/_4$ cup

Yogurt, nonfat, sugar-free, 1 cup

Fish/Seafood (all preparations except fried)

Bass, 2 ounces

Clams, steamed, 10

Cod, 2 ounces

Crab, 2 ounces

Flounder, 2 ounces

Grouper, 2 ounces

Halibut, 2 ounces

Lobster meat, $^1/_2$ cup

Oysters, without shells, $^1/_3$ cup

Pollack, 2 ounces

Salmon, 2 ounces

Sardines, 2 ounces

Scallops, 2 ounces

Shrimp, 5

Snapper, 2 ounces

Squid, 2 ounces

Swordfish, 2 ounces

Tuna, canned, packed in water, 2 ounces

Meat

Bacon, Canadian, 2 long slices or 2 thin, round patties

Bacon, Canadian, extra lean, 3 long slices or 3 thin, round patties

Bacon, turkey, 2 long slices

Bacon, turkey, extra lean, 3 long slices

Beef, chuck, roasted, lean only, 2 ounces

Beef, bottom round, all fat removed, 2 ounces

Beef, eye of round, all fat removed, 2 ounces

Beef, ground, extra lean only, 2 ounces

Beef, round tip, all fat trimmed, 2 ounces

Beef, top loin, all fat removed, 2 ounces

Beef, top sirloin, all fat removed, 2 ounces

Ham, baked, lean only, 2 ounces

Lamb chop, loin, lean only, 2 ounces

Poultry

Chicken breast, not fried, 2 ounces

Turkey breast, ground, 2 ounces

Turkey breast, not fried, 2 ounces

Tofu

Soy crumbles, $1/2$ cup

Tofu, baked or grilled, 2 ounces

Veggie burgers (like Boca Burger), 1 original-size burger, $3/4$ of bigger varieties

Fats

Fruits

Avocado, mashed, ¹/₄ cup

Nuts

Almond butter, 1 flat tablespoon
Almonds, whole, 14
Brazil nuts, unblanched, 4
Cashew butter, 1 flat tablespoon
Cashews, dry or oil roasted, 11
Chestnuts, European, roasted, ¹/₄ cup
Filberts/hazelnuts, 11
Macadamias, roasted or dry roasted, 5 nuts or 1¹/₂ tablespoons
Mixed nuts, dry or oil roasted, 2 tablespoons
Peanut butter, 1 flat tablespoon
Peanut butter, reduced fat, 1 flat tablespoon
Peanuts, dry or oil roasted, 20 nuts or 2 tablespoons
Pecans, dry or oil roasted, 7 halves or 2 tablespoons
Pine nuts, dried, 2 tablespoons
Pistachios, dry roasted, 2¹/₂ tablespoons
Pumpkin kernels, dried, 2 tablespoons
Sesame seeds, 2 tablespoons
Sunflower seeds, dry or oil roasted, 2 tablespoons
Tahini (sesame butter), 1 flat tablespoon
Walnuts, black, chopped, 2 tablespoons
Walnuts, English, chopped, 8 nuts or 2 tablespoons

Oils

Canola, 2 teaspoons
Corn, 2 teaspoons
Olive, 2 teaspoons
Peanut, 2 teaspoons
Safflower, 2 teaspoons
Soybean, 2 teaspoons
Soybean/cottonseed, 2 teaspoons
Sunflower, 2 teaspoons

Salad Dressings/Sandwich Spreads: Save calories and save a fat serving by using nonfat salad dressings and nonfat sandwich spreads. If you limit these nonfat dressings to 4 tablespoons, you will still have a fat serving to spare.

Blue cheese, low-calorie, 6 flat tablespoons

French, low-calorie, 6 flat tablespoons

Italian, low-calorie, 12 tablespoons

Italian, regular, 1 1/2 tablespoons

Mayonnaise, imitation, low-calorie, 2 1/2 flat tablespoons

Mayonnaise, regular, low-calorie, 2 1/2 flat tablespoons

Ranch, low-calorie, 3 flat tablespoons

Tartar sauce, low-calorie, 3 flat tablespoons

Thousand Island, low-calorie, 4 flat tablespoons

Vinaigrette, 1 1/4 tablespoons

Vinegar and oil dressing, 1 1/4 tablespoons

Vegetables

Olives, all types, 20

The following snacks are healthy alternatives to chips, in the portions listed. Each contains one carbohydrate serving and one protein serving and makes a great snack.

Campbell's, low-sodium

Chicken with Noodles, 1 cup

Chunky Vegetable Beef, 1 cup

Split Pea, 1 cup

Health Valley, no salt added

Organic Lentil, 2 cups

Split Pea, 1 3/4 cups

Health Valley, salt added

Black Bean and Vegetable, 1 1/2 cups

Italian Minestrone, 2 cups

Lentil and Carrots, 2 cups

Split Pea and Carrots, 1 3/4 cups

Pritikin: All varieties except Vegetarian Vegetable, which doesn't have enough protein, 1 1/2 cups

Sushi: Avocado and cucumber roll made with brown rice (6 pieces)
Note: Count 6-piece brown rice sushi roll as 1 "always" carb,
³/₄ "friendly" fat, ¹/₄ veggie serving.

Soy chips, 30 chips (This includes 1 "sometimes" carb and
1 "thumbs-up" protein.)

Still feeling hungry after a snack? Fill up on all of the veggies you
want (with the exception of peas, potatoes, and corn) as long as you
don't add oil, fatty salad dressings, or another fat source.

EIGHT

Where There's a Will, There's Water

Myth Busters

MYTH: You always can tell when you are dehydrated because you feel thirsty.

BUSTED: Your thirst is not an accurate indicator of whether or not you are hydrated. In fact, by the time you feel thirsty, you are already dehydrated.

MYTH: You should always drink an electrolyte replacement drink like Gatorade when you exercise.

BUSTED: Unless you are exercising intensely for an hour or more, you need to drink only water to keep you hydrated. Drinking a caloric drink like Gatorade could backfire, giving you more calories than you actually burn through your exercise, negating any weight-loss benefit you get from the exercise.

TIP

WASH YOUR WATER BOTTLE. If you reuse a plastic water bottle, be sure you wash it daily, using plenty of soap. Saliva is a breeding ground for dangerous bacteria.

We are both generous when it comes to sharing food, but when it comes to her sports water bottle, Tammy is stingy.

We cannot overstate what an important role water plays in our metabolism and health. And when exercising, we both realize that without water, we would be unable to work out as long and as hard as we need to.

When we tell clients that Tammy doesn't share her water, they laugh and say that Lyssie can have some of theirs. They also say that before they came to see us they would have thought that Tammy and I were crazy. Many of them could not understand how anyone could drink the recommended minimum eight glasses of water a day, let alone more. However, after several weeks with us, they too became water fanatics. People who could barely swallow just one glass of water a day are easily drinking eight glasses a day. Gone is their lethargy, weight gain, water retention, afternoon headaches, and quickly aging skin.

First, let us tell you the story of one particular client. We taught a weight-loss program in Atlanta where participants met with us once a week for ten weeks. John was unable to make it to the weekly meetings until the end of the third session. Luckily for John, it was not too late for him to start firing up his metabolism.

John's only goal for the week was to increase his water intake. He typically drank only 1½ glasses of water a day; his goal for this week was to aim for 6 to 8 glasses a day. He was to carry around a water bottle all day, reminding him to drink. John far exceeded our expectations; he actually drank more, 10 glasses a day. That was the only change John made in his diet, and one week later he arrived at class *seven pounds lighter!* As you can see, drinking water is a surefire way to help you lose weight. We're going to explain how water works in your body so that you can see how John was able to lose all of this weight, and you will be able to also.

The Power Potion Is Water

Most of us take water for granted. We can get it almost anytime and almost anywhere. Yet, ironically, we rarely have any interest in actually drinking it. People are willing to pay for vitamin "potions," powders, and weight-loss aids that claim to benefit the body in many ways when, as it turns out, water produces many of these very same benefits. The great news is that drinking water won't leave a hole in your pocket and it doesn't come with the dangerous side effects that many of the "potions" and powders do.

TIPS

SQUIRT LEMON, SQUIRT LIME. AS LONG AS YOU SQUIRT IT IN WATER, YOU'LL BE JUST FINE. If you hate the taste of water, this may be just the trick to get your body hydrated and your metabolism revved. Plus, you'll get some extra vitamin C.

VITAMIN WATER—SAVE YOUR PENNIES. Don't rely on water with added vitamins or herbs to give you the nutrients you need. Often the amount of vitamins or herbs in the water is close to nil, and some herbs can be dangerous. So get your vitamins from the food you eat and, if you want to, take a multiple vitamin supplement. But don't bank on that fortified water being your supplement.

Our Twin Trial

in which we show how water washes away extra pounds

Tammy: I couldn't believe I lost the coin flip again. I tried everything in my power to persuade Lyssie to be the guinea pig and drink only three eight-ounce glasses of water a day, despite the fact that she had won the toss. I even accused her of cheating. I swore that she must have weighted the penny in her favor—how could it always land on whatever she called? In one last, desperate plea, I even begged, "This time it's my turn to toss the coin into the air." Sadly, Lyssie reminded me that I had actually tossed every coin flip for these guinea pig experiments.

So the experiment began. Surprisingly, there was good news—day one and only two trips to the bathroom . . . all day! This was a huge decline from my ten to twelve trips a day. I guess that is what happens when you cut back from drinking more than a gallon of water a day. Unfortunately, that is where the good news ended. For starters, I realized that all my years of experience finding the best bathrooms in so many cities was now useless. What good is the knowledge that in New York City on the south side of Central Park the cleanest bathroom is at the Plaza Hotel, when you don't even need to use the bathroom?

In addition to my three glasses of water, I was allowed two other calorie-free beverages per day. I was consuming the same amount of fluid as the average American. I decided that I would drink one glass of my allotted water in the morning, a diet soda with lunch, and a diet soda with dinner. I would save my other two glasses of water for my exercise session.

I always wake up parched, and I must say that eight ounces of water upon awakening didn't quench my thirst. My body was accustomed to awakening and eating breakfast while drinking almost four times this amount! Suddenly, I couldn't wait for my morning exercise so that I could drink more.

It was during this experiment that I began to notice a trial theme: The guinea pig always seemed to be short on energy. From the very first day of the water experiment, my energy level at the gym dropped. On several occasions I had to cut my workout time, as I was exhausted or light-headed or just overheated. Making matters worse, after I completed my exercise, I had a hard time recovering. All day long I felt exhausted, and it was difficult for me to focus. I always felt thirsty, and I developed a late-afternoon headache nearly every day. My skin felt dry and my lips were chapped. Could all of these ill effects be the result of dehydration? Yes. My urine was dark yellow and scarce, another sign that my body was dehydrated.

Unfortunately, my husband, Scott, cued me in to another negative consequence of this trial. He said that he held off two weeks into the trial, but he couldn't take it anymore. Apparently, ever since the first day, my breath had become *far* from pleasant. (I am putting this lightly.) I had been completely unaware of this—I mean, sure, my mouth was dry, and bad breath does accompany a dry mouth, but it just didn't occur to me that my dehydration would play such a role in the smell of my breath. As Scott told me the news, I felt humiliated and instantly had flashbacks to the people I had spoken to (and may have offended) in the last two weeks. The faces flashed by so quickly that I nearly lost my breath in mortification.

At the end of the four-week experiment, it was time to see the results. I weighed myself, and I was two pounds heavier. However, remember that the human body can be up to 60 percent water, so a lot of weight can be lost due to dehydration. In reality I would soon see how much weight I really gained when I wasn't dehydrated. My body fat percentage was the true measure, and it increased by 3.7 percent. This was probably due to the fact that my energy level was significantly impaired and I wasn't able to exert as much effort at the gym or during the day for everyday activities, and thus I wasn't able to burn as many calories. This, in turn, slowed my metabolism and contributed to the increase in my body fat percentage. Two days after the experiment ended, I returned to my normally well-hydrated self and was four pounds heavier than before this experiment began. However, within one month of returning to my normal, water-drinking self, I lost the four pounds.

How Can Water Help Me to Fire Up My Metabolism and Shed Pounds?

The benefits of water are highly underrated. Every single process in your body takes place in water. Every cell is filled with water and every chemical reaction relies on water. This includes the essential chemical reactions that take place so that your body can produce energy, allowing you to be active, burn calories, and have an efficiently running metabolism. Every movement, from the blinking of your eyes to the stimulation of a nerve to riding a bicycle, requires energy, which cannot be produced without water. If simple movements, such as raising your finger or getting up out of your chair, are not performed because dehydration has made you too tired, your inactivity will cause your metabolism to slow significantly.

If you have ever experienced tingly fingers and/or toes when exercising, dehydration may be to blame. The water available in your body is primarily being used to carry oxygen to your working muscles to help you to perform your exercise. When you are dehydrated, this leaves very little bodily fluid to carry oxygen to your extremities. The tingling results from a shortage of oxygen in the hands and feet.

If your body doesn't get the water it needs for its chemical reactions, your metabolism is affected in another way. Since water is a component of your blood, which carries nutrients and oxygen to your organs and extremities, you need enough water in your blood to deliver the nutrients to every cell so it can survive. Your metabolism relies on a well-functioning body. Without enough water you pay the price in a slower metabolic rate.

There are many other ways that water is necessary for a fully powered metabolism and fat loss.

Your body needs oxygen in order to make energy. Without abundant water in your blood to carry oxygen to your muscles, you are sluggish and less active, and you burn fewer calories. What's more, without enough water, the foods you eat and their vitamins, minerals, and other nutrients cannot be efficiently shuttled to sites throughout the body and therefore do not benefit your body to their maximum potential. This means that some food is not turned into usable energy.

Other Ways Water Aids Fat Loss and Continues to Fire Up the Metabolism

Water fills your stomach. Drink a large glass of water before a meal or a snack, or when you're hungry, and we guarantee that you are less likely to overeat and will consume fewer calories when you eat solid food. We encourage you to bring a water bottle with you wherever you go. You are much more likely to drink water if it is always with you. Drink plenty of water with meals as well; water helps fibrous foods to expand in your stomach and fill your belly. (Think of a sponge that expands when it is soaked with water.) You will notice that you feel full more quickly.

Drown Your Hunger

A number of our clients mistake thirst for hunger. That's right, sometimes when you think you are hungry, your body is actually thirsty. Clearly, if you've gone without eating for a long time, this is not the case. However, when you are on our Fire Up Your Metabolism plan, and you feel hungry in between meals and snacks, you may actually be experiencing thirst. So the next time you feel hungry between meals/snacks, drink a tall glass of water to determine if your feeling of hunger is actually coming from thirst.

Our client Hal was waking up ravenous every night around 3 A.M. Hal would wander down to his kitchen and prepare a peanut butter and jelly sandwich and a large glass of milk, and sometimes he'd have cookies, too. When Hal tried drinking water upon awakening in the middle of the night and found that the water "quenched" his hunger, a better night's sleep was not all he received in return. In the first week alone, he dropped 4½ pounds! You, too, can have great results by first drinking water when you feel hungry to figure out if your hunger is actually generated by thirst.

TIPS

CAN THAT CAFFEINATED COFFEE. Although you may feel as though coffee is helping to hydrate you, you are actually losing about half of the fluid you drink. Caffeine acts as a diuretic, allowing you to absorb only about 50 percent of the fluid.

SIP GREEN TEA, BUT DON'T ADD MORE THAN A TEASPOON OF SUGAR. Green tea is loaded with cancer-fighting antioxidants, and several studies have indicated that it can give your metabolism an extra boost. Be aware that green tea contains caffeine, so you don't absorb all of the fluid you drink.

The Benefits of Water Pour on and On

Water is one of the few beverages that are calorie free. This is more important than you may realize. When you drink beverages that contain calories, such as juices, Gatorade, soda, milk, wine, or mixed drinks, your brain does not compensate for these calories later in the day by feeling less hungry and wanting less food, as it does when you *eat* calories. Instead, you continue to eat the same amount of food, while drinking calories, and this can lead to weight gain.

The consumption of simple sugars found in soda and fruit juices wreaks havoc on the metabolism. When you eat a sugary food or drink, your blood sugar rises quickly, causing the body to release a high amount of insulin. Insulin shuttles the sugar from the blood to the muscles to keep blood sugar levels constant. This is your body's normal, natural, and healthy response after eating a sugary food. However, this surge of insulin leaves the blood low on fuel, therefore needing a quick energy source. (See Chapters 2 and 3 on carbohydrates for a complete description.) At this time, your brain is signaled that your body needs more energy and fuel; so you turn to food to provide energy, and you consume excess calories. Clearly, this can cause weight gain.

On the other hand, when you drink water, you get zero calories and your brain does not get the urgent signal that you need more food. Therefore, no excess calories.

Many of our clients have lost weight by simply cutting juice out of their diet. Jessica ate a very healthy diet with an abundance of fruits and vegetables, and she exercised daily. She also drank orange juice and apple juice several times throughout the day. She lost eight pounds in one month—and the only change she made in her diet was replacing the juice with water.

V8 SPLASH—VEGGIES IN A DRINK? It's only 25 percent real juice. The rest is sugary water. Skip it.

NIX SODA—UNLESS YOU'RE LOOKING TO CRASH. After consuming 150 calories of pure sugar per can, your body will have to kick out extra insulin to remove the overwhelming amount of sugar from your blood. You will be left with very little sugar in your bloodstream, and your brain will receive the signal that it needs more fuel. You'll turn to another quick-energy source, such as a candy bar, to provide you with the boost.

DIET SODA IS OKAY. Not great. Not terrible. Just okay. Choose it only occasionally, as it provides your body with fluid but doesn't cleanse your kidneys as water does.

GULPING GATORADE? BETTER NOT. Unless you're a serious athlete or are exercising intensely for more than an hour, you are getting too many unnecessary calories.

Other Beverages That Benefit Health and Metabolism the Same Way Water Does

Although some other beverages do provide a few benefits of water, they do not provide all of the benefits. If you refuse to drink water, and drinking another beverage is the only way you will get fluid, then go and get fluid.

Your best option after water is seltzer. Add a twist of lemon, lime, or orange for zest. Seltzer is calorie free and 100 percent pure. Water is a better choice because seltzer's bubbles may cause gas or bloating, causing some people to limit their consumption and, therefore, not meet their fluid needs.

Teatime. It is always a good time for tea! Drink it before a meal to help satiate you. Just be sure to choose a decaffeinated tea or an herbal tea without added sugar and one that doesn't contain caffeine before bed so you'll be sure to get your z's.

Water has even more benefits over other beverages, including 100 percent fruit juice. You see, your kidneys must filter all of the nutrients, vitamins, and minerals you eat. This means that your kidneys are working very hard all day long. Water is the only way to cleanse and flush out your kidneys. So although 100 percent fruit juice has many vitamins that are important for you, your kidneys still have to filter these nutrients. Your kidneys are like a coffee filter, which water easily passes through. Now imagine pouring sugar on the filter. The sugar will just sit there, piling up. Very little, if any, sugar will pass through the filter on its own. This is why water is essential; when you pour water on the sugar, the sugar passes through the filter, cleansing it. Your kidneys work similarly.

New research indicates that although all fluid consumption is important to your health, water consumption in particular has a beneficial effect on childhood and adult obesity; your overall health as you age; your risk of urinary stone disease and cancers of the breast, colon, and urinary tract; mitral valve prolapse; and salivary gland function. Also keep in mind that caffeinated coffee, tea, and soda do not help to hydrate you as much as you might think; the caffeine they contain acts as a mild diuretic. For example, if you drink an eight-ounce cup of coffee, you are not providing your body with a full eight ounces of hydrating fluid; you are providing your body with only about four ounces. Therefore, you do not get the same metabolic boost that you would receive from a full eight ounces of water.

If it doesn't say "100 percent juice," it's not, and you can count on getting mostly sugar from the beverage. Don't be fooled by fruit drinks such as Fruitopia that say "100 percent vitamin C per serving." Flavors such as Strawberry Passion Awareness and Tremendously Tangerine contain 5 percent strawberry and a whopping 95 percent fructose corn syrup, which is really just sugar.

Most people's kidneys lose much of their capabilities as they age. By cleansing your kidneys with water, you help to keep them in good condition.

TIP

FORGET ABOUT BOTTLED WATER. You're better off using a filter such as the Brita filter on your faucet. Often bottled water is taken directly from the tap, and the water that is bottled from lakes or springs has no real advantage.

Will Drinking Water Make Me Bloated?

Many clients say they don't drink water for fear of bloating. They believe that if they are bloated they should stay away from water because it will make them look and feel worse. This is a *big* myth. Water actually *prevents* bloating. When your body doesn't receive enough water,

Eat your fruit and drink your water. This way you reap all of the benefits of the fiber, vitamins, minerals, and even the cancer-fighting compounds of the whole fruit without all of the unnecessary calories that can accumulate in a serving of juice. (Juice concentrates the calories from fruit in just a small serving.) You will also feel fuller from eating the fruit, especially if afterward you drink water.

it feels threatened as though it may not receive more, and it holds on to whatever water it can. For example, if you eat a lot of salty foods, receptors in your brain stimulate you to drink. If you don't drink, your body tries to maintain its acid-base balance by holding on to all of your stored water to dilute the salt. The result? Bloating. However, if you drink additional water to dilute the sodium, your body returns to a normal sodium-to-water ratio. At this point, your kidneys respond by excreting extra sodium and water together. And that's when you become bloat free. Refraining from water actually backfires in combating bloating.

TIP

EAT YOUR WATER. Foods contain water, too! Fruits and vegetables can be up to 95 percent water. Meat products contain very little water and don't contribute to your body's water needs. So load up on fresh fruits and vegetables.

What Time of Day Should I Drink Water?

Drink water consistently throughout the day. Your body relies on water for every reaction in the body, all day long.

Water and Exercise

During exercise, most of us become thirsty, and this is an excellent opportunity to take advantage of your thirst. However, it is important to realize that the thirst response is actually blunted during physical exercise. Many studies have shown that most exercisers don't drink enough to replace the water they lose during activity. During exercise, the body uses more water for all of its physical processes, not just for perspiration. Water carries nutrients and oxygen to working muscles, moistens lungs to facilitate breathing, lubricates joints, and of course regulates body temperature and cools the body through sweat.

Therefore, it is crucial to drink an additional four to eight ounces

As a bonus, water prevents your skin from sagging after weight loss. Have you ever noticed someone whose skin appears to be hanging loosely from his or her body after losing a large amount of weight? Well, if that person with "loose skin" drank more water, it would fill the spaces between the cells and help to prevent the skin from sagging.

of water for every fifteen to twenty minutes of regular exercise and eight to ten ounces for every fifteen to twenty minutes of extremely strenuous exercise. Follow the guidelines below.

- *Before exercise:* At least 16 ounces

- *During exercise:* At least 4–8 ounces every 15–20 minutes

- *After exercise:* At least 24 ounces

Grabbing a sip of water every so often from the water fountain isn't good enough. To make the most of your metabolism, bring a water bottle with you when you exercise. If you don't like using a water bottle with a pour spout, then use a water bottle with a straw. Some people find them less cumbersome.

There is no excuse for not having a water bottle when exercising at the gym. However, we do realize that in certain situations, perhaps when running outside, it is not practical to carry one. In those situations, grabbing sips of water from available water fountains is certainly better than not drinking at all. Your best option may be to invest in a CamelBak, a backpacklike water bottle that has long, flexible straws that reach to your mouth. (For more information, go to www.camel bak.net.) For your best protection, make sure that you drink enough throughout the day so that you aren't dehydrated when you start your exercise. Then, as soon as you finish your activity, be sure to drink eight ounces of water for every twenty minutes you exercised. Be especially vigilant on hot or humid days—you need to drink even more then.

It is imperative to realize that the one thing that prevents you from

There is an exception to the water rule: Although it is rare, there is the possibility that you could overhydrate. If you exercise for an hour and a half or more, plain water may not be your best choice, as you need to replace electrolytes lost through sweat. In this case, try a drink like Gatorade or, better, a low-calorie electrolyte-replacement drink.

exercising efficiently is drinking too little water, which in turn has negative effects on your metabolism. According to the *Journal of the American Dietetic Association*, dehydration of as little as 2 percent loss of body weight results in impaired physiological and performance responses. You will not be able to focus or exercise nearly as hard or as long as you could if you were well hydrated. Therefore, the boost your metabolism gets from exercise is decreased, and the post-exercise metabolic boosting effect is blunted too (see Chapter 10).

TIPS

YES, PELLIGRINO AND SELTZER COUNT, EXCEPT BEFORE EXERCISE. Pelligrino and seltzer both provide your body with needed fluid and are great drink options—except when you are exercising. The bubbles in these beverages are made from carbon dioxide, and when you are exercising, you are already fighting to rid your body of carbon dioxide and exchange it for much-desired oxygen. So at this time it is not a good idea to take in more carbon dioxide.

DRINKING RED BULL TO GET YOU "FIRED UP"? The only thing you'll be "upping" is your sugar intake and your caffeine intake.

How Do I Know If I'm Hydrated?

Many people are dehydrated and don't realize it. Our clients often ask us how they can know if they are properly hydrated. We always offer these words of advice: Check your urine. If you don't drink enough water, your urine will be extremely concentrated and it will be dark and scanty. When you are adequately hydrated your urine will be pale or clear. Until then, you need to keep drinking. Sixty-four ounces of water a day is usually enough to hydrate the average person. Be aware that if you take vitamin supplements, your urine will be darker for a couple of hours after taking the vitamin as you are voiding the excess that your body doesn't use. At this time you are better off using the volume of urine as an indicator rather than the color. You want to make sure that you have plenty of volume. The bottom line: If you are frequenting the toilet only once every four to five hours, you are dehydrated. On the other hand, if you are running to the bathroom every hour, you may be overhydrated.

What About Alcohol?

Before we ruffle anyone's feathers, let us first tell you about the benefits of alcohol when you drink it *in moderation*. Alcohol, in moderation, can improve your ratio of good to bad cholesterol and it can reduce your risk of heart disease. If you are a red wine lover, there is more good news for you. It appears that red wine, in moderation, may lower your risk for some kinds of cancers. So the bottom line is that when it comes to health, alcohol can be beneficial in moderation.

What is "moderation"? For women, moderation means one drink or one serving of alcohol per day. For men, it means two servings per day. Here are "servings":

- Wine, 5 ounces
- Liquor, 1½ ounces
- Beer, 12 ounces

Bear in mind that more than one drink per day for women and two drinks per day for men can have negative effects on every system in your body.

Which alcoholic beverages are the worst? The drinks likely to add the most calories are mixed drinks that contain sugary fruit syrups or sodas.

FRUIT JUICES AND SODA DON'T MIX WELL WITH MIXED DRINKS. They add hundreds of extra calories to an already calorie-dense drink. When you have a cocktail, the calories in the drink mixes and juices can exceed those in the actual alcohol.

How Does Alcohol Affect My Metabolism and My Weight?

Research conducted on twenty-six men by the University of Dundee in Scotland showed that when the men drank alcohol and then ate a meal, they increased the amount of calories they consumed by 30 percent; they didn't seem to compensate for the excess alcohol calories by eating less. In fact, it appeared that alcohol might even stimulate the appetite. Unfortunately, this excessive consumption of food and alcohol bogs down the metabolism as the body fights to deal with such a large amount of calories. Remember, your metabolism especially suffers from a large calorie intake if you have not eaten for a while, because your body can't deal with all of the calories while it is in "conservation mode" and it readily stores the excess as fat. (See Chapters 6 and 7 for a complete explanation.) For example, this happens when you arrive at a cocktail party, happy hour, or dinner—long after you've eaten your last meal.

A study published in *Nutritional Neuroscience* offered more bad news: After drinking alcohol, people actually take longer to feel full from food, and alcohol consumption also makes you feel hungry sooner—a double whammy!

Alcohol also dehydrates your body and, as previously discussed, this slows your metabolic rate. In addition, alcohol blocks Acetyl-

CoA, an important molecule that is necessary in order for your body to create energy. This means that Acetyl-CoA is unable to reach your body's energy-producing cycle and, instead, Acetyl-CoA molecules become building blocks for fat (fatty acids). Meanwhile, your body is left sluggish and deprived of energy, resulting in a depressed metabolic rate as your body has less energy to perform everyday movements.

Alcohol also disrupts the functioning of your liver. It is the liver's job to package fatty acids (triglycerides) so that they can be sent out of the liver. When alcohol is present, the liver has to stop its usual job and break down the alcohol, as your body must rid itself of this harmful toxin. So fatty acids accumulate (fat accumulation on the liver can be seen after a single night of heavy drinking). As you can imagine, a liver clogged with fat cannot function properly, which results in liver damage.

Alcohol causes the acid in your body to rise, creating a dangerous and sometimes life-threatening situation. Too much acid in the blood (called acidosis) causes proteins to lose their shape; this renders them useless. To give just one example, hemoglobin (a component of your red blood cells), which is made up of a protein, loses its capacity to carry oxygen throughout the body. The result of acidosis can be a coma and even death.

NINE

Sleep Satiated Versus Sleep Starved

Sleep deprivation leads to intense sugar cravings, the inability to feel full after eating plenty of food, impulsive eating and compulsive overeating, decreases in lean muscle tissue, impaired ability to obtain energy from carbohydrates, and a decrease in physical activity.

Myth Busters

MYTH: An alcoholic drink before bed helps you to sleep better.

BUSTED: Alcohol is a depressant, so initially it may help you to feel more relaxed and tired, and help you fall asleep. But after it's metabolized it has a rebound and stimulatory effect and can make for a very restless night, causing wakefulness. Depressants such as alcohol disrupt REM sleep. Scientists are still trying to discover exactly why this happens. So avoid alcohol for at least three hours before bed.

MYTH: The only bad thing about not getting enough sleep is feeling tired.

BUSTED: When your body doesn't get the sleep it needs, everything is affected negatively, including the speed of your metabolism.

Eight hours of sleep seems like a colossal waste of time, doesn't it? After all, we live in a time-crunched society where every minute is precious. Instead of spending hours sleeping, we could take advantage of this time to respond to E-mails, take a yoga class, spend time with friends and family, or even hit the spa. In fact, some clients and friends are proud to say that they are so busy and have so much to do that they try to sleep only a few hours a night so that they don't miss anything. Some of these live-life-to-the-fullest people have even told us that sleep is for the "weak." Well, this is all very superhero-like, but it's not conducive to healthy living or to weight loss and a speedy metabolism.

Our Twin Trial

in which we show that increasing your sleep increases your metabolism

In all our previous trials, the guinea pig who did not follow our Fire Up Your Metabolism principles experienced a recurring sensation— plummeting energy levels. And the guinea pig inevitably wound up slowing her metabolism and gaining weight. So in this trial, when the loser would have to be sleep-deprived, we expected the result to be tiredness and slowing of the metabolism.

Our sleep-deprivation theory was that the guinea pig's metabolism would be slowed immensely by sleep deprivation, resulting in substantial body fat gain. First, we suspected that the lack of sleep would cause her to be exhausted and have no energy to be active—even small movements would be difficult; therefore, she would burn fewer calories, slowing her metabolism.

Second, we anticipated that the sluggishness and slowing of the metabolism would be exacerbated, since sleep deprivation damages your ability to metabolize carbohydrates, your body's favorite fuel.

Third, we believed her metabolism would be impaired, as the production of important hormones, including growth hormone, would be reduced. As you will learn in this chapter, growth hormone helps you to build lean muscle mass, thus speeding up your metabolism. Remember, the more muscle you have, the more calories your body burns, so we were expecting the guinea pig to lose some muscle and therefore slow her metabolism as less growth hormone is produced from a body that is lacking sleep.

Finally, we anticipated that the sleep-deprived twin would gain weight because she would make a common mistake. Her body would be craving energy, and therefore she would misinterpret this as her body's cry for fuel, causing her to eat.

Tammy: I lost the coin toss. While Lyssie had three months of utter bliss, enjoying eight hours of sleep a night, I was allowed only a mere five and a half to six hours of sleep a night. While Lyssie awoke refreshed and rejuvenated every morning, I awoke to the awful buzzing of my alarm clock. Day after day, for three months, I dragged myself out of bed, cranky, eagerly awaiting nighttime so that I could go to bed, only to be reawakened, still tired, still cranky. (I would like to thank my wonderful husband, Scott, for putting up with his grouchy wife.)

Do I sound a bit bitter? In three months, Lyssie slept approximately 207.25 hours more than I did, but who's counting? And the worst part about my three months of misery, aside from feeling absolutely dreadful is that my metabolism slowed because it was suddenly hard to resist unhealthy snacks. During this trial, we allowed my usual diet to be altered so we could see any effects of sleep deprivation on food choices. However, I was still trying to use my usual restraint.

It wasn't long after the trial started that I found myself in a state of complete and utter exhaustion. I had *no* energy, *none.* Getting up out of my chair felt like a chore. This was completely new to me, as I had never even noticed getting up or moving before. Now, even little movements were a struggle. I was leaning on desks, countertops, and walls when I was standing up. My body was attempting to save some energy, because it didn't have much left.

The good news was that throughout the entire first week of this trial, I was temporarily relieved from my feelings of exhaustion during my morning exercise routine. I did have to push myself to get my butt to the gym, but once I got started exercising, it was the one time of the day that I seemed to have a little more energy; I didn't remember that I was sleep deprived at all. And looking back on this trial now, I think that forcing myself to exercise, which got my blood flowing, was the best thing I could have done for myself. However, I admit that by the second week and throughout the remainder of this trial, my cardio workouts felt more challenging than they usually did, and I couldn't exercise as intensely as before. To my surprise (and chagrin), my strength decreased, too. I could no longer lift the weights I once could. So I have to admit that when I was feeling exhausted, my only motivation to get to the gym was that the cardio would help to wake me up!

Since I felt lifeless and was moving little during the course of the day, I was gradually slowing my metabolism. My exhausted body was craving a big rush—an immediate surge of energy. I was desperately searching for simple carbohydrates such as jelly beans, gummy bears, or any other sugary snack I could get my hands on. The worst part about it was that on days when I gave in to my cravings and after consuming far too many "useless" sugar calories and experiencing the debilitating effects of a "sugar crash," the reality set in. I was never actually hungry in the first place; I simply was tired and really craving energy. Also making matters worse, as the sugar crash started to take place, my body yearned for yet another energy boost; I craved another quick pick-me-up. I tried to resist these cravings with every bit of strength that I could drag out of my exhausted body; I desperately wanted to avoid getting caught in a vicious cycle, which is hard to do when you are not rested.

So how did sleep deprivation affect my metabolism? The result of our twin trial devastated me. My body fat increased by 4.2 percent, which meant I had gained 4.4 pounds of body fat. I am only five foot three, so 4.4 pounds is not easy to hide! After all, this meant I had gained 5 percent of my total weight, which is nothing to sneeze (or in this case, yawn) at.

I was thrilled that I was heading for a full night of uninterrupted z's. Although usually quite a night owl, that night I hit the sheets at 9 P.M. and slept for a full eight and a half hours. I awoke feeling refreshed and alive, something I hadn't felt in several months.

How Much Sleep Is Necessary to Have a Speedy Metabolism?

If you're like most people, your body requires at least eight hours of sleep to provide for sixteen hours of sustained wakefulness. If you're like the average adult, you are sleeping only about six hours a night, and you are falling far short of your body's sleep requirements.

TIPS

CATNAPS JUST FOR KIDDIES? NOT A CHANCE! Short daytime naps replenish energy and keep you alert.

ONE THING IS SURE TO BACKFIRE—EATING BEFORE BED. Although eating large amounts of food promotes drowsiness, as much of your body's blood and oxygen supply rushes to your stomach, leaving your muscles and brain to compete for the remaining blood supply, eating large amounts of food before bed is counterproductive. When you are lying down, it can cause indigestion or an upset stomach that can wake you up in the middle of the night.

DROWN IT OUT. Noises frequently disrupt a sound night's rest. By using a fan or a white noise machine, loud neighbors and busy street noises are barely detectable, and you can have a sound and uninterrupted night's sleep.

KICK THAT RECLINER TO THE CURB! Falling asleep on that ole recliner or couch while watching late-night TV may feel good at first, but it rarely leads to a full night's sleep. Find a comfortable bed and fall asleep there!

Sleep Deprivation—What a Doozy

When your body doesn't get its needed sleep, the negative results are practically endless. For starters, your body actually stimulates a chronic inflammatory response; this is a prolonged inflammation that occurs when your body is trying to protect itself from injury. Although an inflammatory response is essential for protecting tissues when you are hurt or sick, chronic inflammation has been shown to damage healthy tissue. Obviously, this is worrisome, as it affects your lifelong health; this chronic inflammatory response is linked to heart disease, high blood pressure, and diabetes. And although these problems may not develop until after the accumulation of many years of sleep deprivation, don't expect that it will take you that long to notice the other ill effects of skimping on your z's.

You are affected right away. You immediately notice daytime drowsiness—reaching for an extra cup of coffee in the midmorning, yawning several times throughout the midafternoon, dozing off during an evening movie. A less obvious result of drowsiness accompanying sleep deprivation is feeling exhausted and thus burning fewer calories all day long. You are too tired to exercise, too tired to play with your kids or pets, and too tired to walk (so you take the bus and the elevator, and don't even stand up in your office, using your office chair with wheels to shuffle around and make life in the "tired lane" easier). So you sit still, not moving a muscle, and barely burn a single calorie.

Adding to this calorie-hoarding bonanza and making "weighty" matters worse, cortisol, a hormone that regulates your appetite, is affected when you are sleep deprived. As a result, when you lose sleep, you may still feel hungry even after you have eaten an adequate amount of food. Additionally, growth hormone, a protein that regulates your body's proportions of fat and muscle in your adult years by helping you to build lean muscle mass and thus speeding up your metabolism, is significantly reduced when your body is deprived of its quality deep sleep. This is critical. Muscle burns calories, so if you don't have enough growth hormone to help you build muscle, your metabolism will drastically slow.

Tired = Inefficient Use of Carbs?

The effects of sleep deprivation don't end there. When you are sleep deprived, your ability to use your body's favorite fuel, carbohydrates, becomes impaired. Sleep deprivation interferes with the body's ability to metabolize carbohydrates, causing high blood levels of glucose. Excess glucose promotes the overproduction of insulin, which may lead to an increase in body fat (not to mention that it can also harm your health by leading to insulin resistance, which often leads to diabetes). However, when it comes to your metabolism, you may remember that carbohydrates provide your body with the only fuel the muscles can store as energy and the only fuel the brain can use as energy. If your body can't use carbohydrates efficiently, it can't get energy, and your health suffers. And when your health and energy suffer, your activity level does, too, lessening the calories you burn and ultimately slowing your metabolism.

TIPS

DON'T BE LATE FOR YOUR "SLEEP APPOINTMENT." Make a sleep appointment with yourself and write it down. Schedule a time that you can get at least eight hours of sleep, and then drop everything else a half hour before your sleep appointment so that you have time to relax and crawl into bed for a sound slumber. You wouldn't schedule a doctor's appointment and then miss it, would you? Well, you shouldn't miss your sleep appointment either.

MIDNIGHT RUMBLING? Eating too little can result in middle-of-the-night awakenings from rumblings of hunger. So if midnight stomach rumblings awaken you, be sure to have a *small* evening snack an hour or so before retiring. See our Snack Lists on pages 168–176 for ideas.

WHO KNEW? VACUUMING AND DUSTING CAN MAKE YOU SLEEP BETTER. Dust and pollen cause breathing difficulties and congestion that may keep you awake. Vacuuming and dusting can keep these sleep disturbers away. A bonus: You'll burn a few extra calories in the process.

RESTFUL ROUTINES—GO TO BED AND WAKE UP AT THE SAME TIME DAILY. As odd as it seems, your body actually has its own "clock," and in order to have the best and most restful sleep, it is important to set your internal clock by going to bed and getting up at the same time every day—even on weekends.

WHEN IS A LITTLE SPICE NOT SO NICE? For some people, spicy foods and highly seasoned foods cause heartburn and indigestion that make falling asleep difficult, if not impossible. For that matter, any food intolerances will interfere with a good night's rest.

YOUR MATTRESS MATTERS. Is your mattress more than ten years old? Does your mattress have a deep groove imprinted where you sleep? Are you achy in the morning? Can you feel the coils in your mattress? Do you sleep better in a bed other than your own? If you answered yes to any of these questions, your mattress may be interrupting your precious sleep. It's time for a new one.

NAPPING AFTER 4 P.M.? DON'T. It will make it too hard to fall asleep at night and will mess up your normal sleep schedule.

TIPS

DON'T DO IT IN THE BEDROOM! Watch TV, that is. Separate television and the bedroom, as a late night with Jay Leno or David Letterman may make you miss out on your critical z's.

CRAVING COOKIES? If you didn't get enough sleep last night, your body is actually craving sleep. Grab a nap, not a cookie.

SAY YES TO A LITTLE BUBBLY BEFORE BED. We're talking about a warm bubble bath! Or try a warm shower or Jacuzzi. They tend to relax your muscles and raise body temperature. So when you get out of the bath, your body temperature begins to drop, which encourages delta sleep (the sleep during which body recovery takes place).

TICKTOCK, TICKTOCK . . . DON'T WATCH THE CLOCK! Watching the clock or dwelling on sleeplessness backfires and causes anxiety and stress, thus keeping you awake.

BE REGULAR ABOUT YOUR EXERCISE. Engaging in regular physical activity makes it easier to fall asleep and stay asleep, and you kill two birds with one stone (see Chapter 10).

HAVING TROUBLE WITH YOUR MEMORY? LACK OF SLEEP MAY BE TO BLAME. It's between the sixth and eighth hours of a night's sleep that the brain really stores everything it learned during the day— habits, actions, and skills. Clearly, your memory and learning ability suffer if you don't get continuous sleep for eight hours.

YOU SAY YOU'VE BEEN FLIPPED MORE THAN A BURGER? If you have spent more than ten minutes flipping, tossing, and turning, get out of bed. Do something low-key. Try reading while you keep the lights low. But don't engage in any activity that is strenuous or anxiety provoking.

LOW-MOTION TRANSFER . . . WHAT'S THAT? Make sure that you select a mattress with it. Low-motion transfer mattresses are constructed so that the coils are not yoked together across the top and bottom. Otherwise, wherever your partner goes, you go, too, which can cause you to lose up to 20 percent of delta sleep.

PICTURE YOURSELF ON THE BEACH. Feel the cool breeze on your skin and the warm sun on your back. Use visual imagery, meditation, or muscle relaxation techniques to reduce stress as much as possible.

FIGHT OSTEOPOROSIS AND SLEEP BETTER. Take one 500-milligram calcium supplement before bed. Not only does calcium fight osteoporosis, it also relaxes your muscles, helping you to sleep more soundly.

I Thought I Was Craving a Cookie, but I Really Was Just Craving a Nap

Adding to this dreary situation and making matters metabolically worse, the body often confuses being tired with being hungry. When you are sleep deprived, your body is having trouble efficiently using carbohydrates so it craves them even more, desperately searching for energy. Thus, you turn to food to give you that boost. The problem is that when you want an instant burst of energy, chances are you don't crave healthy carbohydrates like whole grains, fruits, and veggies. Instead, you crave the carbohydrates that provide the quickest pick-me-up.

That of course, is sugar, a "rarely" carbohydrate. Candy bars, chocolate, cookies, and cakes—these are the foods to which most sleep-deprived people turn.

TIPS

LIGHTEN UP! Put on your sunblock and head outside for some sunshine. Sunlight, especially in the afternoon, helps to reset your body's clock. Research shows that night-shift workers can improve daytime sleep by working under bright lights.

THREE-WAY LIGHT DIMMERS ARE FOR MORE THAN JUST ROMANCE. One-half hour before bed, set the dimmer on its lowest setting and make the ambience more soothing. The dim light will help you to relax and transition to bedtime.

KEEP YOUR CLUTTER IN YOUR CLOSET—LITERALLY. Keep your clutter out of your bedroom. With the clutter out of sight, you won't stress about what you need to do, and this will make for a peaceful night's sleep.

SILK ISN'T NECESSARY. Try 100 percent cotton sheets. They're comfortable, durable, cool, and soft. They'll help you to fall into a deep slumber.

YOUR HEAD IS NO PLACE FOR YOUR WORRIES AND STRESS. LEAVE THEM ON YOUR DRESSER. Stress often disrupts a good night's rest. You toss and turn and can't get your brain to shut up. A few hours before bed, jot down your stresses and anxieties and ideas for solving the most pressing problems and leave the list on your dresser. This will take your mind off your problems, as you now have possible solutions for them.

DO YOU HAVE ALLERGIES? ARE YOU SENSITIVE TO CHEMICALS? Pure-finish sheets and allergen-resistant pillows and bedding may be your new best friend. All traces of chemicals are removed, or the sheets are made without chemicals at all, which means no allergens and better sleep.

CREATE A WINTER SLUMBERLAND. Use a humidifier. Dry air can make your skin itchy or cause respiratory problems. A humidifier moistens the air and makes you comfortable and ready for a good night's sleep.

YOUR COLD OR ALLERGY MEDICATION COULD BE KEEPING YOU UP. Who knew that taking it several hours before bedtime could disrupt your sleep? Medicines such as Sudafed and Drixoral frequently cause sleeplessness and could keep you up, so avoid them before bed.

What's more, something else may be contributing to these carbohydrate cravings, causing an even more intense and more profound yearning for sugary and fatty carbohydrates—low levels of a brain chemical called serotonin. Serotonin enhances a general sense of calm and positive feelings, and it seems to be recharged when your body rests. This means that if you are lacking rest, you have low serotonin levels, which result in craving that positive mood as well as foods that are rich in carbohydrates (and often full of fat). Therefore, in order to prevent craving sugary and fatty calorie-laden treats, protect your serotonin levels by getting adequate sleep.

Another way to keep your serotonin levels up is by eating adequate—not excessive—amounts of carbohydrates and moderate amounts of protein. Diets that contain too much protein can interfere with serotonin production, ultimately disrupting calm and positive feelings.

TIPS

WHAT? DID SOMEONE SAY EARPLUGS? Yes. These aren't soundproof but will shut out sounds from noisy neighbors or a mate who snores. Disruptive noise can make getting a good night's rest virtually impossible.

AAAAAAH! BREATHE DEEP. Try this deep-breathing technique if you are having problems falling asleep. Breathe in through your nose for four counts, hold the air in your lungs for seven counts, and breathe out through your mouth for eight counts. Repeat three times. This stimulates your parasympathetic nervous system, which in turn slows your heart rate, causing rest, relaxation, and sleep.

SQUEEZING IN YOUR EIGHT GLASSES OF WATER AT THE END OF THE DAY? You do need that water, but try to get it in earlier in the day, as adequate fluid intake reduces fatigue while enhancing relaxation. If you overload on water just before bed, you are likely to have to make several overnight visits to the bathroom.

MEDICATE A HEADACHE BEFORE BED? BETTER NOT. At least not with Excedrin Migraine, Anacin, Cafergot, Fiorinal, and Fioricet, as they all contain caffeine and will keep you awake. Instead, try Advil, Tylenol, or another caffeine-free painkiller.

DON'T SLEEP WITH YOUR PETS. Half of the people surveyed in a Mayo Clinic–conducted study said their pets disturbed their sleep.

TEN

Fidgeting, Frolicking, and Keeping Fit

Myth Busters

MYTH: As long as you exercise, it doesn't matter if you sit around the rest of the day.

BUSTED: Although exercise is important for your weight and metabolism, if you sit on your butt whenever you are not exercising, it will negatively affect your weight and slow your metabolism.

MYTH: If you consistently run five miles a day, you will definitely see results.

BUSTED: Running five miles is significant and can help you to stay in shape while allowing you to eat more food and still maintain your weight (or lose weight). However, if you consistently run five miles every time you exercise, your body will eventually become accustomed to the run, and the results will plateau. If you want to get stronger, fitter, and leaner, you need to change your workout either by mixing up the speed during your run, or changing your exercise completely, so that your body is challenged. Different muscles will be activated and you will burn more calories.

MYTH: Some people are just lucky and don't have to exercise.

BUSTED: Although some people are lucky and look good on the outside without having to exercise, on the inside they may look terrible. Exercise is critical for good health. Your heart is your most important muscle, and if it isn't worked regularly, it will be in bad shape.

MYTH: If you exercise, you don't have to worry about what you eat.

BUSTED: Although you can eat more calories in order to maintain your weight, your diet is only half of the equation to a lean and fit body. Exercise doesn't make up for a poor diet loaded with fatty foods that clog your arteries. If you frequently eat foods such as bacon, fast-food burgers, and cookies, even if you exercise, your body may look okay, but your arteries will still look bad.

Our Twin Trial

in which you learn why even the little movements really do matter

Our clients often ask us if they really have to exercise. They ask, "Can't I fire up my metabolism by just changing my diet?"

Although you can fire up your metabolism by following our eating guidelines, what you eat is only part of the equation. Exercise is the other part of the equation, a critical factor in revving up your metabolism to your ultimate potential.

In this trial, we wanted to see just how much our exercise routine and our active lifestyle affected our metabolism and our weight. Since we exercise extremely consistently and are always on the go, we expected the results of this trial to be fairly dramatic.

Lyssie: This time I lost the coin flip. I wasn't allowed to perform cardiovascular exercise for two months. In addition, I had to cut back on my "fruitful frolicking"—this means I had to force myself to sit down and stay seated at times when I normally would be walking around or standing up while talking on the phone, cleaning my apartment, cooking dinner, doing laundry, getting dressed, putting on my body lotions and makeup, brushing my teeth, or painting my nails. At first, I was so accustomed to moving all about that I kept forgetting to sit still. In fact, I grew worried that I would wreck this trial if I didn't chain myself to the couch.

However, I discovered an enjoyable way to deal with this restriction—I started taking *long* relaxing bubble baths. While soaking, I talked on the phone, read magazines, or listened to the radio. I would sit in the bath for hours, and when I was so pruned that I looked like an old lady, I knew I had done my job.

I tried to be optimistic. I thought, "Okay, I'll have more free time to involve myself in other activities and I'll still eat as healthfully as always, which of course will help me feel great."

For the first couple of days I enjoyed my newfound "free" time. Instead of going to the gym to do my cardio, I caught up on correspondence with friends and got things done, things that I never seemed to have time to do—going to the post office and the bank, picking up pharmacy prescriptions, and getting my hair highlighted and my nails manicured. However, within a couple of days, this free time disappeared. I'm not sure where it went. After several weeks, I found myself growing antsy and impatient more quickly than usual, especially when I was feeling stressed. I became irritated about the smallest things, like my mom on the phone confusing my voice with Tammy's and calling me Tammy. (This is something we usually laugh at.) I wasn't sure why this was happening. I figured it was because I wasn't alleviating any stress at the gym, or taking out my aggressions from a rough day on the treadmill.

I later realized that one reason I was irritated was that my pants were feeling uncomfortably tight, and although I wasn't consciously aware of it, the pressing on my stomach was making me uncomfortable and it was causing me to be short-fused.

I also noticed that I didn't have much of an appetite. I would have never thought this would be a bad thing, but I guess I take having a good appetite for granted. Not having an appetite is how I feel when

I am sick. I never realized how much healthier you feel when you have a good appetite.

Needless to say, when the two-month trial was over, I was ecstatic. I couldn't wait to get back to the gym, return to my normal energy level, get my "runner's high," and fit comfortably into my pants again. In fact, instead of waiting until the next morning to get back on track with my normal exercise routine, I would go to the gym that night.

I was in for a rude awakening. First, when I went to put on my exercise top, I noticed that the skin around the tank top in the back puckered out around the elastic. Also, my stomach protruded. I was horrified. I had felt heavier, but I hadn't realized how much my body had changed. After twenty minutes of trying on different workout outfits, I threw on a huge T-shirt that nearly hung to my knees. I then forced myself to go to the gym. Walking there, I prayed that I wouldn't see anyone I knew.

When I got to the gym, I refused to make eye contact with anyone as I quickly hopped on the treadmill—the one in the corner, where no one could see me. Little did I realize that I was in for my second rude awakening; I completed my jogging warmup and ran for only two minutes before I felt breathless and exhausted. I tried to push on at my old pace, but I felt completely winded. I was forced to slow the treadmill and eventually wound up jogging for my entire workout at the speed I usually use for walking during my cool down. I couldn't believe I had been away from the gym for only two months. I was so discouraged that I cried as I walked home. I knew that I had a long way to go before I got back into shape.

So just how much does exercise and "fruitful frolicking" affect my metabolism? *Significantly.* This trial, as we suspected, affected my metabolism more than all other trials. The two-month trial resulted in a whopping 6.3 percent increase in body fat, which was a six-pound body fat gain. The amazing part was that I was eating just as healthfully as I always do, and less food, due to my reduced appetite.

Exercise's Uplifting Benefits

Having a bad day at work? Woke up on the wrong side of the bed? Fighting with your significant other? Physical activity is the perfect medicine to lift your mood. When you are physically active, your body releases endorphins, "feel-good" chemicals that make you feel euphoric.

That's not the only reason to perform physical activity. Exercise helps you fight heart disease, high blood pressure, diabetes, and many other diseases, as well as helps you lose weight by speeding up your metabolic rate.

The best news is that you don't have to wear yourself out and exercise like a maniac to experience most of the benefits of exercise and increase the amount of calories you burn daily. You should, in fact, be able to hold a conversation while you exercise, making it a great activity to do with a friend, which prevents boredom. (However, if you can sing, then you aren't challenging yourself enough and you need to pick up the pace.)

Calories Burned . . . Burning . . . and Still Burning?

Everyone knows that physical activity burns a lot of calories while you are doing it and thus fires up your metabolism. In fact, our friend Julie tells us that although she doesn't *love* to exercise, she does it for the love of her favorite foods.

Even after you've stopped exercising and are sitting on your couch or in your office chair, the metabolism-revving benefits of exercise are still working. This novel thought seems too good to be true—accelerate the rate at which you burn calories as you exercise and then burn extra calories and fire up your metabolism even after you've finished. You see, when you exercise, your body increases the speed that it burns calories (your metabolism speeds up). When you stop exercising, your metabolism is still revved, so it continues to burn calories at an increased rate for some time. Visualize it this way: Your metabolism is like a slow-burning fire. Exercise for your metabolism is like wood for the fire. Adding wood helps the fire to burn harder, just as exercise gets your metabolism to burn more calories. And even after you stop adding wood, the fire continues to burn more intensely for quite some time. Likewise, even after you exercise, your body continues to burn calories at a faster rate for a while.

Exercise moderately every day and the *after*-exercise calorie burn can be about thirty-five calories, accumulating to about 3½ pounds of fat loss per year. Strenuous daily exercise can enable you to burn as much as 180 extra calories after you stop, which can add up to eighteen pounds of fat loss a year.

There's more good news. All physical movement can burn calories and fire up your metabolism. Most people know about cardiovascular exercise, which really gets your heart pumping and involves moving large muscle groups over an uninterrupted period of time (such as running, biking, or swimming). We call this "cardiovascular contentment," and it is very beneficial when it comes to your metabolism because simply doing it requires your body to burn up more calories. (Remember, your metabolic rate is the speed at which your body burns up calories. Since "cardiovascular contentment" makes your body burn more calories, it increases your metabolic rate.)

TIPS

CANCEL YOUR LAWN SERVICE. Mow your lawn yourself and burn 225 calories for each half hour you mow. Use your push mower on your lawn while walking at a brisk pace for more than an hour and you can skip cardio that day.

JUMP FOR JOY. Performing sets of jumping jacks not only burns calories and speeds up your metabolism, it also releases your body's feel-good chemicals, sending you into a euphoric state.

SNAZZ IT UP! Invest in some trendy exercise clothes—you'll be motivated to exercise simply by being eager to wear the snazzy clothes.

GET INTO THE SWING OF THINGS. Take a swing class with a friend—learn how to dance while getting your heart pumping.

THE FALL SEASON MEANS LEAVES FALLING OFF TREES AND POUNDS FALLING OFF YOU. Make a habit of raking your yard daily. You will have the cleanest lawn on the block and the speediest metabolism.

BE A KID. Play soccer or tag in the backyard with your kids. No kids? Bring out the kid in you by indulging in childhood games— make a snow angel or play hopscotch.

JUMPING ROPE? YOUR METABOLISM HAS NOTHING BUT HOPE. Jumping rope is one of the best ways to fire up your metabolism and burn mega-calories. The average-size person will burn about two hundred calories in fifteen minutes.

PUT EVERY MUSCLE IN YOUR LEGS ON MAXIMUM ALERT. Mix up your walking/jogging pace. Alternate sprints with slower bouts to accelerate your toning results.

WALKING FAST CAN BE MORE CHALLENGING THAN JOGGING. That's because you've got to push harder to speed up. Squeeze your inner thighs to pump up your pace and your toning.

"Cardiovascular Contentment"

Cardiovascular exercise or, as we like to say, "cardiovascular contentment," requires a large group of your muscles to move over a sustained period of time. Swimming, biking, walking, running, aerobics, hiking, skiing, in-line skating, dancing, playing active sports, and any other repetitive activity that can be performed over a long period of time all qualify as "cardiovascular contentment." (Ever taken a "cardio-striptease" workout class? This, too, qualifies.) So even if you have tried to get in shape before and have been unsuccessful, this time you can choose a new exercise that is enjoyable. Now is the time to be active. You will never feel better and you'll never be so fired up.

If you are like most of our clients, even after you have read the previous paragraph, you are still wondering which exercise is the best, or which exercise machine you should use to burn the most calories. Does the stationary bike or the cross-trainer machine burn more calories? (One cardiovascular machine does not burn more calories than another. It is how much you challenge yourself— the more you challenge yourself, the more calories you'll burn.) The machine you like better is the one you should use. If you like something, you're more likely to do it and stick with it. If you don't like the exercise you are doing, you may get burned out and skip several sessions of "cardiovascular contentment." But make no mistake about it: Even your least favorite exercises are enjoyable if you listen to your favorite music or talk to your friend while you exercise. Those endorphins will kick in and you will begin to feel the euphoric effect.

TIPS

BETTER SOME THAN NONE! No excuses! Even five minutes of cardiovascular exercise burns more calories than nothing at all. Don't use time as an excuse—even if it means arriving at your front door after work and walking ten minutes in one direction and then coming back home.

SPLIT IT UP! Exercise can seem much more exciting and much more doable if you don't spend all of your time doing the same thing. For example, if you are aiming for thirty minutes of cardiovascular exercise, try ten minutes on the StairMaster, ten minutes on the treadmill, and ten minutes on the cross-trainer. When you exercise for only ten minutes on each machine, there is light at the end of the tunnel—not to mention that you work more muscle groups and benefit from cross-training.

SKIPPING ISN'T ONLY FOR KIDS. Burn extra calories by picking up the pace of your walk—skip.

DO IT JUST FOR KICKS. Kickboxing is a great way to rev your metabolism, burn extra calories, shape your lower body, and to get out some aggression. Enroll in a class near you.

DO IT BACKWARD. Getting bored with your walking workout, need a variety? Get yourself to a track and walk as quickly as you can—backward! You'll use muscles that you haven't used before. Just be careful to watch where you're going.

PUT A SPRING IN YOUR STEP! Jump and dance on a minitrampoline at home in front of your TV, or take a specialty class at the gym that uses trampolines.

PUNCH OUT YOUR AGGRESSION. You don't have a punching bag? Take your pillow and punch it as hard as you can for five minutes. You'll get your heart pumping, and you'll be amazed how great you feel after you've punched out your pillow and it doesn't hit you back.

How Do I Know If I Am Exercising with Enough Intensity to Fire Up My Metabolism?

The key to getting the most out of your workouts is making sure that your heart rate is in your target heart rate zone. Staying within this zone enables you to exercise for a long period of time while ensuring

If you are a beginner, don't aim for a THR of 70 or 80 percent in the hope of speeding up the process. This won't make you look better faster. It will just cause exhaustion and muscle strain (and maybe injury), perhaps preventing you from exercising for several days.

that you are working out intensely enough to get real results, firing up your metabolism to its ultimate potential. It is safer to exercise at a mild to moderate intensity than a more vigorous intensity. But if you exercise too mildly, you won't get the metabolism-revving results you are looking for.

Your target heart rate (THR) is the number of times your heart should beat per minute while you're exercising. First determine your maximum heart rate (MHR): Just subtract your age from 220. Your THR depends on your age and fitness level. If you are a beginner, or if you are trying to exercise longer or harder, your THR should be 60 to 70 percent of your MHR. If you are at an intermediate fitness level, your THR should be 70 to 80 percent of your MHR. If you are at an advanced level of fitness, your THR should be 75 to 85 percent of your MHR.

We've done the math for you. Use the Target Heart Rate table below. Find your age, then find the percent that is right for you.

Target Heart Rate

TARGET ZONE (THR)

Age	MHR	60%	70%	80%
20	200	120	140	160
25	195	117	137	156
30	190	114	133	152
35	185	111	130	148
40	180	108	126	144
45	175	105	123	140
50	170	102	119	136
55	165	99	116	132
60	160	96	112	128
65+	155	93	109	124

You should aim to get your heart rate into your target zone every day for at least a half hour. If you can do it for longer, say, an hour, you will fire up your metabolism even more.

In order to determine your heart rate, you need to feel your pulse. You can find it on your wrist (radial pulse) or your neck (carotid pulse). To find your *radial pulse,* use your middle and pointer fingers—not your thumb—to locate the pulse on the thumb side of your wrist. Press lightly and count your pulse for fifteen seconds, starting with zero. Multiply that number by 4 to get your rate per minute. Keep exercising while taking your pulse, just move at a slower pace. To find your *carotid pulse,* place your thumb on your chin. Swing your pointer and middle fingers onto the side of your neck. On each side of your neck, there is a groove. Feel for your pulse. Do not press both sides of your neck, and don't press to hard. Count for fifteen seconds, starting with zero. Multiply by 4.

TIPS

CALLING ALL SHOPAHOLICS. Find the largest mall you can. Walk around the mall three to five times before entering a store. After each store, make another loop around the mall. It will give new meaning to the phrase "shop until you drop."

HANGING ON FOR DEAR LIFE? DON'T. If you are using an exercise machine, don't hold on too tightly. Putting the machine on a high level, only to hang on to the machine, results in fewer calories burned, because the machine does more of the work.

YOGA AS YOUR ONLY FORM OF EXERCISE? THINK AGAIN. Although all forms of yoga are good for your mental health and will help improve your physical strength, most forms of yoga don't require you to move muscle groups repetitively for a sustained period of time, nor does your heart rate stay elevated long enough to count as your daily "cardiovascular contentment."

WORKING OUT IN THE MORNING TO BURN MORE CALORIES? NOT NECESSARILY. Although a few studies have shown that some

people achieve a slight edge in metabolic boost after morning workout sessions, your metabolism will be increased for several hours after a workout no matter what time of day you exercise. Exercise when you have the most energy, because you will be able to exercise more intensely, leading to a greater after-exercise metabolic boost. (Keep in mind that if you exercise first thing in the morning, your exercise won't be pushed to the side as other engagements take precedence over your afternoon or evening exercise sessions.)

GARDENING ISN'T ONLY FOR THE ELDERLY. Gardening can be quite challenging and can really help you burn extra calories and rev your metabolism. You'll burn about 185 calories per half hour of gardening.

FORGET ABOUT CAR WASHES. Do it yourself and rev your metabolism by burning more than one hundred calories in a half hour.

DANCE THE NIGHT AWAY. You'll have so much fun that you won't even realize that you're burning about one hundred calories for each fifteen minutes of dancing.

WHO SAID KNITTING WAS ONLY FOR GRANDMA? Knitting is the perfect thing to do when watching television. It burns a few more calories than just sitting there doing nothing. Not to mention that your hands will be occupied and unable to be used for snacking, as many people engage in mindless eating and consume far too many calories while sitting in front of the TV.

Think the Little Things Don't Matter? Think Again

Although you should engage in a half hour to an hour of "cardiovascular contentment" *every day*, the little things you do ("fruitful fidgeting and frolicking") can make an enormous difference. You've heard it before: Very small activities such as taking the stairs instead of the elevator are beneficial to health and in weight loss. Clients have remarked, "I mean, really, how much will it really help my weight-loss efforts to take the farthest spot in the parking lot or to take the stairs instead of the elevator? It just seems like a big waste of time." It's not. Take a peek below and you'll see that the little things you do for exercise are hardly a waste of time.

- Stand for ten minutes every day at a time when you normally sit, and this metabolic jump-start will save you from packing on two pounds this year.

- Get off the bus one stop earlier and walk four blocks to your office every day. You'll get a metabolic boost and burn forty calories. Do it for one year, and that's equal to three pounds. Do the same thing on the way home and now you're talking more than six pounds per year.

- Taking two flights of stairs instead of riding the elevator twice a day will save you almost 1½ pounds per year. Now that's nothing to sneeze at. (And by the way, every time you sneeze you burn a calorie.)

One of our favorite examples of the benefits of "fruitful frolicking" involves one of our celebrity clients. We want to respect her confidentiality, so we will call her Jen. When Jen came to us, she was very lean, yet she was still fighting to lose "those last five pounds" in order to meet the rigorous industry standards of TV and film. Like many of our clients, Jen engaged in forty-five minutes of "cardiovascular contentment" most days of the week. However, when we examined Jen's typical daily caloric intake, we noticed that she was eating almost twice as many calories as our other clients who were about Jen's size and who exercised about as much. Jen was somehow able to maintain a body that was as lean as, if not leaner than, these clients.

Here's how. During the day, most of our other clients are fairly inactive. Jen spends long days on the set. She is constantly on the go. She is standing much of the day and realized while she was in our office that she rarely even takes a breather to sit down. It turned out that Jen can eat so much more food than other people her size and with similar cardiovascular routines because she burns twice as many calories from her "fruitful frolicking" than from her daily forty-five-minute "cardiovascular contentment" routine.

IN THE OFFICE? Fire up your metabolism by getting out of your office chair and moving around.

LOOK, MA, NO HANDS! Invest in a hands-free headset for your telephone. This will free up your arms so that you can move and groove around the home and office while you talk on the phone. Do this for ten minutes a day at a time when you usually would be sitting down, and you'll burn an extra thirty calories—more than three pounds over a year.

STAND UP FOR YOURSELF! Don't even think about leaning on anything.

GET ON THE BALL! EVEN IF YOU THINK YOU ALREADY ARE. Even get on it while watching TV. Sitting on a big resistance ball forces you to use good posture and burn a few calories from "fruitful fidgeting and frolicking."

WALK THE DOG . . . DON'T WATCH THE DOG WALK. Too many dog owners are guilty of just letting the dog go out the back door. Be sure you join your dog for his walk!

SQUEEZE IT ALL DAY LONG. A hand-size stress ball, that is. Not only is this a great stress reliever, it also helps to fire up your metabolism by burning a few extra calories.

REACH FOR THINGS. Put things that you use frequently on higher shelves so you'll have to reach up to get them. You'll burn extra calories along the way.

LEFT, RIGHT, LEFT RIGHT. That's right, march in place. Sitting at your desk? Lounging on your couch? Every hour get up and march in place for several minutes. It will rejuvenate you.

UNLOAD YOUR GROCERY BAGS ONE BY ONE. Each trip back to the car burns additional calories. Be grateful for heavy packages. The heavier the package, the more calories you burn.

CANCEL THE HIRED HELP TO SHOVEL YOUR DRIVEWAY. By doing it yourself, you not only save money, you also rev your metabolism.

CHANGE YOUR SHOES WHEN YOU GET TO THE OFFICE. Be sure to wear comfortable shoes to the office and then change when you get there. Otherwise, it will be easy to make excuses to take the bus or the elevator rather than to walk or to take the stairs.

NEED TO USE THE RESTROOM AT WORK? Take the stairs and go to another floor and burn some calories on the way. You might even meet new people.

Excused from Your Excuses?

We've heard it all. We know all of the excuses. There are a million reasons why you must lie on the couch rather than engaging in "cardiovascular contentment" or "fruitful fidgeting and frolicking." We've had twenty-five-year-olds tell us they're too old, healthy people tell us they're too sick, energetic people tell us they're too tired, people with all the free time in the world tell us they're too busy, muscular-framed people tell us they're too weak, and slim people tell us they're too fat. No matter what your excuse, simply remember that the benefits of exercise carry far more weight than the comfort of lying on your couch. It is time to do something. And you *can* do it. And you *will* do it. You will start *today*. And we're going to help.

SIT UP ON THE COUCH; DON'T LIE DOWN. Doing this for just two hours a day equals a three-pound fat loss over the course of a year. Go figure.

Converting That Couch Potato into a Spunky Spud

If you are a couch potato, it's time to become a spunky spud and shed a few fat layers. We have a little something that we like to call MAGIC (Motivate, Appointment, Gather friends, Imagine, and Create a reward) that will make exercise part of your routine so that it becomes a habit; your metabolism will be fired up for the rest of your life. Study after study shows that people who lose weight and are best able to keep it off have made exercise a habit, not an on-again, off-again activity.

M = Motivate. Start by motivating yourself. Keep a pen and a piece of paper next to you for the next couple of days and write down every reason you have to exercise. Include reasons such as being able to fit into all of the clothes in your closet, feeling attractive enough to date, seeing more muscle tone in your arms, looking good at your high school reunion, wearing a bathing suit this year at the beach, feeling comfortable in public, relishing walking up the stairs without feeling breathless, improving your health, increasing your energy, being able to live a long and healthy life, having more energy to spend quality time with your family, etc. Keep this list by your pillow. If your motivation to exercise ever starts to wane, use this list to remotivate yourself.

Now set some goals, which will motivate you. Just keep in mind if you've never performed physical activity, you can't expect to enter a marathon by next week. You must start slowly and gradually build up your stamina. But do set a lofty goal for yourself. You *can* run a 5K. And if you start training now, you *will* be able to run a marathon within a year. (And when all else fails, think about this: A 150-pound couch potato uses up only about one calorie per minute while sitting on the couch—that's only $1/280$ of a Snickers bar.)

Keep an exercise journal (on the log below). It, too, will serve as a motivator as you watch your stamina improve and see how far you've come. Track every move you make from the very beginning. Include the times you take the stairs instead of the elevator, when you do jumping jacks in front of the television, etc. Be invigorated by all of your improvements, as every change, even the smallest one, makes a huge difference over your lifetime.

Exercise Journal

TARGET HEART RATE RANGE: _____ (see page 216)

Date	Total Minutes	Type of Exercise	Heart Rate	Comments

Next, motivate yourself by making it official. Tell your family, friends, and colleagues that you are going to start exercising consistently, for the rest of your life. Put a sign on your refrigerator. Your goal is to make exercise official and commit to yourself.

Last, always remember that *you are in charge of your body,* and only you are responsible for taking care of it. No one else can or will do it for you. *You control you.* No one can take away your achievements, but no one can make you exercise, either.

A = Appointment. Set a time for exercise. Before breakfast? During your lunch break? After work? Put it on your calendar every day, and select a backup time, just in case something interferes with your exercise commitment, such as an important meeting at work. Scheduling a backup time for exercise ensures that your commitment is foolproof. Also, it makes you feel in control of your life, because you know nothing can interfere with your plans to take care of yourself and your weight. By setting an appointment, you'll be taking a proactive approach to speeding up your metabolism.

Make this exercise appointment part of your routine, like brushing your teeth. For us, heading to the gym for our morning exercise has become a habit. We get up, wash our faces, put on our exercise clothes, eat breakfast, brush our teeth, and head to the gym. We don't even think about doing it—or not doing it—we just do it.

G = Gather friends and make it fun. It sounds simple, but if you don't make exercise enjoyable, you are less likely to do it. This may mean listening to music or a book on tape, or even watching TV while exercising. Maybe you bike or walk to your favorite store.

Try a team sport, or an exercise class, where exercise is also a social activity. You can hire a personal trainer to help you in your mission. Or find an exercise buddy. This way, when you feel like flaking out of your workout, you will be disappointing someone else besides yourself.

I = Imagine. Imagine yourself succeeding in your exercise routine. Disney said it best: "If I can dream it I can do it." Imagine a new, re-shaped body. Imagine a healthy body, one full of life, vigor, and energy. Carry this mental image with you wherever you go and think of it several times a day. This body can and *will* be yours. Don't allow yourself to get discouraged. Make a list of positive affirmations. They'll help you think positively and help to eliminate negative thoughts. Read these affirmations out loud several times a day. (If someone is around you and saying them out loud makes you feel self-conscious, repeat the affirmations in your head.) Hang them on your mirror and your refrigerator, and put a copy in your wallet.

Here are a few suggestions for your list. (Make your own list tailored to your lifestyle.)

- I need to exercise so that I am confident enough to date.

- I am going to eat a healthy afternoon snack so that I am not hungry after work. Instead I can go to the gym rather than home to eat.

- Aside from my normal exercise, I am going to start making many little movements throughout the day, such as always walking around when I talk on the phone, getting up and moving around during television commercials, and sitting up straight so that I will lose ten pounds and look great by the time of my sister's wedding.

- I will go for a half-hour walk five days a week so that I can stay off cholesterol medication.

- I am going to go for an hour bike ride every afternoon when I get home from work because I need to feel comfortable in my clothes.

- I am no longer going to dislike myself. This self-loathing needs to stop. I need to feel good about myself, so I am going to take a spinning class every day after work.

- Every day I am going to get off the bus four stops earlier and walk the rest of the way because I want to get my morning off to a good start so that I can feel in control of my day.

- I will make a pact with my friend to meet her every morning to go for a walk because I need to lose weight so that I will look good when it is time to put on my bathing suit for my vacation.

- I'm going to take an aerobics class four times a week because I need to lower my blood pressure.

- I will walk and jog with my treadmill on an incline, rather than flat on the ground, because I want to look great—just for me.

C = Create a reward for yourself. Reward yourself every month. Your gift to yourself could be anything—treating yourself and a friend to a healthy dinner or to a massage, buying a new pair of running shoes or, better yet, new pants (you will need a new pair anyway, as your old ones will be too big). You have dedicated yourself to a wonderful cause, bettering yourself and improving your health. You deserve a reward.

What If Exercise Is Already a Habit?

Many clients who walk in our door for the first time are already exercising regularly. All too often, they come to us out of frustration; they exercise several times a week, consistently, yet can't seem to lose the extra weight. For example, Melvin was running for forty-five minutes on the treadmill five times a week. At first he lost weight, but after six months, the scale wouldn't budge below 185. He ate sensibly, but even that didn't have an effect. His annoyance and frustration were growing.

Melvin's body had become accustomed to his run, which is why it was no longer a challenge for him. Melvin's running routine had helped him lose weight and now was enough for him to maintain that weight, but not for him to see more results. Here's why: When you continually do a certain exercise, your body uses the same muscles all of the time, and they are no longer challenged—they move so efficiently that they actually conserve calories, causing your body to burn fewer than you once did when the exercise was a challenge for you. It was time for Melvin to "shake things up a bit" so he could "shock" his body and fire up his metabolism.

We put Melvin on an interval-training program. Melvin was to continue running, as always, five days a week. For three out of those days, though, Melvin would not run at his typical 7-mph pace; instead he would start by running for three minutes at 6 mph. Then he would increase his speed by 1 mph, every minute, for three minutes. So, after running for three minutes at 6 mph, he would run at 7 mph for a minute, then increase his speed to 8 mph for one minute, and then to 9 mph for a minute. After that he would recover for three minutes at 6 mph. He would repeat this cycle—called intervals—until he had run for his usual forty-five minutes. Melvin would not be accustomed to this new and more challenging exercise regimen, and his body would have to burn more calories.

Melvin was shocked and pleasantly surprised when he realized how much he enjoyed the interval training. He couldn't believe how quickly his run "flew by." Six weeks later, Melvin had dropped seven pounds. The interval training had kick-started his metabolism. Interval training caused him to reap other benefits—his usual five-mile run at 7 mph had become surprisingly easy, and he started to pick up the pace of that running routine.

Melvin became ambitious: He wanted to return to his high school

Short, high-intensity exercise periods alternated with low-intensity recovery periods can fire up your metabolism. The higher-intensity exercise will challenge your body in new ways and you will burn more calories, as you will have to activate more muscles for the new challenge.

weight of 165 pounds and asked how he could fire up his metabolism even more. "Cross-training," was our reply, a method of physical training in which a variety of exercises or modes of exercise are used to stimulate additional strength gains and reduce the risk of injury. We suggested that Melvin try using the cross-training machine two times a week and the StairMaster once a week instead of running every day. He was already an efficient runner, so new cardiovascular exercises would activate different muscles and challenge his body, burning extra calories. So Melvin began cross-training *and* continued to perform his interval training the other two days of the week. Within eleven weeks, he'd lost another four and a half pounds.

TIPS

UP, UP . . . AND POUNDS MELT AWAY! Walk or run on an incline. Increase the incline on the treadmill and you will burn up to 50 percent more calories than on a flat surface.

DO IT EVERY THREE MINUTES. Whether you are walking, running, or exercising on any machine, turn up the intensity and perform an "ultrapower" high-intensity interval for one minute. Repeat every two to three minutes.

ELEVEN

Muscles Make Magic

Myth Busters

MYTH: If women engage in strength training, it will make them look bigger or bulkier.

BUSTED: Strength training does not have to make you look bigger or bulkier, unless you want it too. In fact, women do not have enough testosterone to create big and bulky muscles. However, women do have the ability to create lean, toned bodies.

MYTH: If you are forty or older and have never lifted weights before, your metabolism has already slowed and it's too late to repair the damage by weight lifting.

BUSTED: Although your metabolism does slow each year after your midthirties if you don't strength-train, it is never too late to reverse this by starting to lift weights. Even people in their eighties who have never lifted a weight in their life can begin to speed up their metabolic rate by strength training.

MYTH: The more you strength-train, the more results you'll see.

BUSTED: Although consistency is definitely a key factor in lifting weights, speeding up your metabolism, and giving results, your muscles actually need rest in order to reap the benefits. You shouldn't work the same muscles two days in a row. Give your muscles at least forty-eight hours of rest.

What if we told you that there was something that will make your body burn more calories while you are still, even when you sleep? What if we told you that this very same thing could make your legs look leaner and tighter and your rear end firm and shaped, and stop the back of your arms from jiggling?

You would probably say, "I thought there were no miracle drugs." Then we would tell you, "You're right, muscles aren't miracle drugs."

Strength training increases your body's lean muscle tissue and, therefore, increases the rate at which your body burns calories. Lean muscle requires many calories simply to exist. So the more lean muscle tissue you have, the faster your metabolic rate, and the more calories you burn all day long. When you increase your lean muscle mass, you fire up your metabolism.

Our Twin Trial

in which we show you why muscles are essential for a speedy metabolism

Lyssie: I lost the coin toss. I was terrified to start this trial. I didn't want to see the results of my years of hard work weight lifting go to waste. I knew what would happen: When you stop strength training, you lose muscle strength, definition, and tone. So we did this trial to see exactly how much I would be affected. Would I gain body fat as I lost muscle? And if I did gain body fat, how much would I gain?

For the first week I enjoyed all the extra time I had. By the third week, any novelty of spare time was replaced by feelings of depression as I noticed that my arms didn't have the muscle definition they used to. And by the sixth week, I told Tammy that this whole trial needed to be called off. Tammy made me stick it out for another two weeks, claiming that we needed to see results. Since I was still doing cardiovascular exercise, I looked thin, but that was it, just thin, not toned. I was what we dietitians call "skinny fat." That is, you look skinny but don't have the low body fat that you appear to when clothed.

At week six, I was truly downtrodden. I had lost strength! I live in New York City, where you can buy only as much as you can carry home. My favorite grocery store is several blocks away from my apartment. I always load my groceries onto the checkout counter and the checkout cashier always assumes that I need to have my heavy bags delivered. I take pride in saying, "I don't need delivery. I'll carry my bags home." Well, on this particular day, I tried my usual bag-carrying routine. My arms started burning so badly that I actually had to stop and put the bags down. I was discouraged, humiliated, and disgusted. Not only was I skinny fat, I was also weak!

At the end of this depressing eight-week trial my clothes felt tight, and although I weighed the same as I had before, my body fat was 3 percent higher than it had been before the trial, which explained why my clothes now felt tight. During this trial I had been eating the same amount of calories I usually eat, and I had been burning off the same amount of calories from my cardiovascular exercise, so the fact that I had gained body fat could mean only one thing—my body was no longer burning calories efficiently and was now storing some calories as fat. The slowdown in my metabolism occurred because I had less calorie-burning muscle. So the food I ate did not get burned off as it usually does. Only part of it was burned off, and I gained fat. My weight stayed the same because body fat took the place of my muscle, and it was the same, pound for pound. My clothes were tight because muscle is denser and takes up less space than fat.

Visualize it this way: A pound of muscle would look compact and dense, like a pager. A pound of fat would look squishy and bulky like the bottom half of a stocking leg filled with cottage cheese. It is evident that you must continue to strength-train if you want to keep your body toned and tight and your metabolism revved.

When Should I Start Strength Training?

Now. Using light hand weights or your own body weight as resistance (push-ups, sit-ups, pull-ups) builds a foundation for muscle tone and a speedy metabolism. After you have laid the foundation for a lean body with adequate muscle tone, your job is easy. Then, it requires only maintenance to keep your metabolism revved.

What Happens If I Don't Strength-Train?

Eventually, as you age, your muscles start to shrink. (Even if you can't see them and you have never exercised a day in your life, muscles are actually there.) As your muscles shrink, dreaded fat takes their place. As you lose muscle, your metabolism starts to slow, and the pounds begin to creep on. If you are a woman, you start losing lean muscle tissue in your late twenties and early thirties. By age thirty-five, you lose $\frac{1}{4}$ to $\frac{3}{4}$ pound of muscle each year and gain that much body fat. The table on page 233 shows how much fat you may gain simply due to aging if you don't start strength training. If you are a man, you start losing lean muscle tissue after the age of twenty-five, with a rate of decline of about 7 pounds per decade, if you don't do anything to halt the process. After the age of thirty, both the size and number of your muscle fibers decrease. Although you may not notice a loss of strength until after you are forty, you actually lose about 5 percent of your strength every decade after that.

What does this really mean? A man who weighs 170 pounds and has 89 pounds of muscle at age twenty-five loses 14 pounds of lean body mass by the time he is forty-five. His metabolic rate declines accordingly, and if his caloric intake remains the same, his body fat increases significantly. After twenty years, he may weigh the same, but he surely does not look the same. See the table on page 233 to learn how many pounds of lean muscle tissue you would lose and how many pounds of body fat you would gain as you aged if you didn't do strength-training exercises.

Women Over Thirty-Five Who Don't Strength-Train

POUNDS OF MUSCLE REPLACED BY FAT EVERY FIVE YEARS DUE TO AGING

Age	Pounds of Muscle Replaced with Fat
Under 35	You may not yet have replaced lean muscle tissue with fat, but you may look flabby in places where you could look lean and toned if you strength-trained.
35	$1/2$–$3/4$
40	$2^1/2$–$3^3/4$
45	5–$7^1/2$
50	$7^1/2$–$11^1/4$
55	10–15
60	$12^1/2$–$18^3/4$
65	15–$22^1/2$
70	$17^1/2$–$26^1/4$
75	20–30
80	$22^1/2$–$33^3/4$
85	25–$37^1/2$
90	$27^1/2$–$41^1/4$
95	30–45
100	$32^1/2$–$48^3/4$

Men Over Twenty-Five Who Don't Strength-Train

POUNDS OF MUSCLE REPLACED BY FAT EVERY FIVE YEARS DUE TO AGING

Age	Pounds of Muscle Replaced with Fat
Under 25	You may not yet have replaced lean muscle tissue with fat, but you may look flabby in places where you could look leaner, more muscular, and toned if you strength-trained.
25	$3^1/2$
30	7
35	$10^1/2$
40	14
45	$17^1/2$
50	21
55	$24^1/2$
60	28
65	$31^1/2$
70	35
75	$38^1/2$
80	42
85	$45^1/2$
90	49
95	$52^1/2$
100	56

Regardless of your gender, you must do something to prevent fat from taking over your body. The vicious cycle must be stopped.

The good news is that there is no need to panic. You can start strength training now and replace fat tissue with lean body tissue. That's right: This vicious cycle *can be* reversed. This means that if you have witnessed undesirable changes in your body with age, you can now feel as though a big, fat burden has been lifted off of you.

We have witnessed this transformation with our clients, from high school students to senior citizens. For example, Jill and Robby had been married for thirty-four years when they came to see us in hopes of losing thirty-five pounds each. Jill was fifty-four years old and going through menopause, and Robby was sixty-four years "young," as he liked to say, just approaching the "best days of his life." Jill and Robby took a half-hour walk together every morning, and they both ate fairly low-calorie diets composed of lots of fruits and vegetables, and adequate whole grains and lean proteins. They avoided sweets and fatty foods. Still, they complained that pounds slowly crept on and body fat shifted to less desirable places. Jill said that she used to have a small waist and an hourglass figure, but now fat seemed to be accumulating on her lower stomach and all around her waist as well as on her back, and she felt "boxy." Robby had looked very athletic in his younger days, but now he felt like he was turning into his father—his legs looked scrawny and his stomach was a protruding "beer gut." Jill and Robby were frustrated; they felt as though they were doing everything right, yet everything about the way their bodies looked— and felt—was wrong.

Fortunately, the problem wasn't a mystery. Jill and Robby were missing an important ingredient in their regimen: strength training.

Recent research at the University of Maryland proved that in only two months of strength training, the average person can recover twenty years of lean muscle tissue loss and three decades of strength loss. Thus, no matter what age you are, you can watch your body become leaner and fitter as you strength-train.

After five and a half months of it, Jill had gone from a size twelve to a size six and lost thirty pounds. Her body had taken on a whole new shape; muscle had replaced so much body fat that Jill didn't even want to lose more weight. She was satisfied with her new lean body. Robby lost thirty-five pounds, and his frail frame had morphed into a muscular one with an almost "nonexistent" stomach. Robby teased that he was going to be the new model for Calvin Klein briefs. Neither could remember ever looking better, not even in their early twenties. Strength training added calorie-blasting muscle to Jill's and Robby's bodies. This allowed them to burn up more calories all day long. Since they were eating the same amount of food as before, their bodies now easily burned up this food and started to burn up some of their fat stores. Also, the muscle they gained was compact and dense. As their bodies shed fat, their newly toned, muscular bodies were revealed.

Now It's Your Turn to Muscle Up Your Metabolism

However, before you get started, it is important to keep in mind that not everyone is the same when it comes to strength training. Some people naturally catch on quickly while others don't. Whatever your strength starting out, remember to progress at your own pace. Don't try to lift something twice as heavy as you can handle just because your friend is lifting that weight. On the other hand, if your friend is lifting a weight that wouldn't challenge you, don't hinder your efforts to turn body fat into lean muscle mass and to fire up your metabolism by working at your friend's pace.

A Pound of Feathers Equals a Pound of Bricks . . . but Does a Pound of Muscle Equal a Pound of Fat?

As you have started to see, although one pound of muscle is equivalent to a pound of body fat in weight, that is where the similarity ends. When it comes to size, touch, and the way they look, body fat and lean muscle tissue couldn't be more different. Fat is large, sprawling, squishy,

If you really like to see numbers to help you to get motivated, there are scales available that measure your percentage of body fat, such as those made by Tanita Corporation at www.Tanita.com.

and it can even look as if it exists in rolls, while muscle is small, smooth, dense, and compact. Visualize it this way: On your body, one pound of body fat on top of your belly looks something like a large balloon filled with Jell-O, while one pound of muscle looks more like a tight, shapely area smoothly covered by the skin of your stomach. (Think back to our twin trial: Although Lyssie weighed the same, she had gained fat and lost muscle, so her clothes were tight.)

So don't judge your progress on the scale; as muscle replaces body fat, the scale may not be a true indicator of just how lean you have become. The way you feel in your clothes is a much more accurate indicator, as you will feel like you are walking on air and your clothes will fit you much better. You may even have to buy new clothes several sizes smaller.

Need Someone to Show You the Ropes?

Although many of our tips don't require that you step foot inside a gym, most gyms offer something that can be invaluable in getting started with your strength training. That *something* is a personal trainer. Although many people don't feel that they need a trainer or don't want to spend the money, we like to think of a trainer as an investment. A physical trainer can actually help you to save money in the long run. A trained professional will teach you exercises that will challenge and strengthen your body while assisting you with your technique. Many trainers will travel to your house; it isn't necessary to belong to a gym. A trainer can warn you and reposition you if you are doing something incorrectly, thereby preventing injuries, doctor bills, and missed work. And, of course, strength-training equipment and exercises seem a lot less intimidating when there is someone to show you the ropes. The good news is that you don't necessarily have to hire a trainer on an ongoing basis (unless you want to); a couple of sessions (sometimes even a single session) can be adequate to get you started on the right foot.

You can ask a health professional or friends and/or coworkers you trust to refer you to a good trainer. Make sure the trainer:

- Has liability insurance.

- Is certified in CPR.

- Is certified in first aid.

- Makes you feel comfortable talking openly and honestly about your weight and goals.

- Has a college degree in an exercise-related field or a master's degree in an exercise-related field and/or a personal-training certification from one of the following reputable organizations: American College of Sports Medicine, American Council on Exercise, Cooper Institute, National Academy of Sports Medicine, National Strength and Conditioning Association, Aerobics and Fitness Association of America.

Your Mission: Molding Your Body into a Calorie-Melting Machine

Your goal is to create lean muscle tissue. Your objective is to strength-train. Your "assignment" is to perform several Fire Up Your Metabolism tips. You can choose a handful of your favorites. For all tips, you will lift the heaviest weight you can (while still maintaining proper form) eight to twelve times; this is one set. If you don't feel challenged by the eighth or twelfth repetition (rep), the weight is too light and you need to increase it. Strength training should hurt. But not so much that you hope Dr. Kevorkian is on the machine next to you. If you can't lift the weight eight to ten times, then you need to use a lighter weight. If the weight is causing you to swing or sway, or if you are not able to keep your body in the correct position, then the weight is also too heavy.

Your first session may take a little extra time as you figure out which weights are the best for accomplishing your ultimate goals. After finding the appropriate weight, you should perform three sets of each exercise, allowing a one-minute rest between each set. (Take advantage of this time to drink some water.) It is important to keep a journal and record the amount of weight that is appropriate for you. It will also help to keep you motivated as you can track your progress and see your strength build.

What If I Have Already Been Strength Training?

You have been building a great foundation for a speedy metabolism. However, remember to keep pushing yourself. Most veteran strength trainers, such as yourself, have figured out their routine at the gym and have become a bit complacent. You may not even really feel challenged anymore. If a day after your workout, you do not feel muscle soreness, you're probably not being challenged enough to really see a difference. So try new exercises, such as the ones below. And although you may be experienced in the world of strength training, it is always a good idea to track your progress; as you see your new strength gains, they will motivate you to continue to increase your weights and to try new routines so that you continually fire up your metabolism. Use the Strength Training Journal on page 239 as your guide.

TIP

STAY ON THE FAST TRAIN BY WAY OF THE CIRCUIT TRAIN. When you circuit-train, you quickly move from one muscle group to the next so you don't use up time waiting for a muscle group to recover. This can help you to be more efficient, as you work more muscles in less time. The key is to minimize your downtime between sets by working opposing muscles. So as you finish a set of hamstring exercises, immediately complete a set of quadriceps exercises, or as you finish a set of biceps exercises, immediately start a set of triceps exercises.

Strength Training Journal

Date	Fire Up Your Metabolism Exercise Performed	Weight Used, in Pounds	Time or # of Repetitions	# of sets	Level of Difficulty
Sample 1/22	Tricep Presses	3-lb. Hand weights	12	3	Challenging
Sample 1/22	Plank Exercise	My body weight	30 sec.	3	Very challenging

Light . . . Lighter . . . Too Light?

Whether you are a beginner or a strength-training veteran, eventually, the weight you are using will begin to feel too light. If you are a beginner, this usually happens after about four to six weeks of training; if you are a veteran, it may happen within a month, as you have probably already experienced this several times in the past. While you have already increased your metabolic rate by creating lean muscle tissue, you are capable of increasing it even more, but you must challenge yourself. It is time to increase the weight you are lifting.

Waiting to Exhale? Don't

When you lift weights, you may find yourself forgetting to breathe. Concentrate on it. Your body needs the oxygen for the working muscles. Without it, energy cannot be produced; you can get dizzy and light-headed, and this could cause you to faint.

Breathe continuously during each exercise, in a relaxed and natural manner. Be sure to breathe out (exhale) during the hardest part of each exercise. For example, if you are doing a push-up, exhale each time you push your body up and away from the ground. As a rule of thumb, exhale when you lift, inhale when you lower. Although it may take a bit of practice, it will become a habit and won't require any attention, just as you breathe naturally.

Should I Lift Weights Every Day?

You shouldn't work the same muscle group every day. When your muscles rest, they recover and build the lean muscle tissue that is essential for firing up your metabolism.

Again, give your muscles a forty-eight hour rest from when you lifted last. So although you could lift weights every day, you would never want to work, say, your triceps two days in a row. You could do a full-body routine three days a week. Or you could strength-train every day, avoiding training the same body part two days in a row. The example below shows how you could train every day but avoid training the same muscle group two days in a row.

Day 1: Legs and abdominals

Day 2: Chest and triceps

Day 3: Back, biceps, and shoulders

Day 4: Legs and abdominals

Day 5: Chest and triceps

Day 6: Back, biceps, and shoulders

Day 7: Rest

For exercising at home, invest in some hand weights. (And you'll get a workout just carrying them home!) A good starter set for women is pairs of two-, three-, and five-pound weights. As you get stronger, you can hold two in each hand for five, seven, and eight pounds. Men may want to begin with ten-, twelve-, and fifteen-pound weights.

In a Time Crunch? Work These Four Major Muscle Groups and Give Your Metabolism a *Real Punch*

Sometimes finding enough time in a day to fit in a strength-training routine that works all the muscles in your body is nearly impossible. But you can get a fabulous, fast workout by focusing on the "big four" muscle groups—the chest, legs, back, and abs—rather than smaller muscle groups, because you are recruiting more muscles and activating a greater number of muscle fibers, thereby burning more calories. The chest, legs, back, and abs make up the majority of your body. Therefore, when you are in a hurry, focus on these muscle groups. Often, when men are in a hurry they focus on their biceps and triceps. In reality, if these men had worked their back and their chest, they would have had a much more productive workout.

Not only do the back and the chest cover a much larger area of the body and cause you to burn more calories then the biceps and triceps, when you work the back and chest you also work the biceps and triceps. Women, on the other hand, tend to work the inner and outer thighs when they are in a hurry, as they want to tone that part of the leg known for jiggling. However, their workout would be more productive if they focused on the larger leg muscles such as the quadriceps and hamstrings (and glutes) rather than the small muscles of the inner and outer thighs.

To make your workout easier, we have divided our Fire Up Your Metabolism tips into different categories: exercises for your back, your abs, your legs, and your chest. You can pick and choose from each group. We also provide tips for the smaller muscle groups so that these can be performed on days when you have more time, or a spare minute in your office, or when you are in front of your television. Remember, although performing exercises for the big four muscle groups is very helpful when it comes to firing up your metabolism, you will have the best results and see the most muscle tone when you include exercises that isolate the smaller muscle groups as well.

TIPS

Abs

PRACTICE PERFECT POSTURE. Standing up straight not only requires you to keep your shoulders back, it also means that you have to keep your abs tight and contracted at all times. If you don't have great abs now, practice perfect posture all day long and soon you will be quite pleased with your own abs!

LET'S BE FRANK. ONE OF THE BEST AB STRENGTHENERS IS THE PLANK. See "Your Strength Training Guide at Home," page 248.

YOU'VE PROBABLY HAD A HUNCH THAT IT'S ABOUT TIME YOU DO THE CRUNCH. This is one of the most effective ways to fire up your abs. See "Your Strength Training Guide at Home," page 248.

HERE'S HOW TO TONE THE FLAB . . . ON YOUR LOWER ABS. Try a reverse crunch. See "Your Strength Training Guide at Home," page 248.

ARE YOU A VETERAN AT THE GYM? THIS AB MOVE WILL HELP YOU GET TRIM. Lie on a physioball. Place your feet on the ground, while your back rests on the ball, parallel to the ground. Follow the directions for performing a crunch ("Your Strength Training Guide at Home," page 248) with the proper technique, and now you are also building your stabilizer muscles!

Chest

KISS THE GROUND . . . IN BETWEEN EACH PUSH-UP. Each peck will make sure that each push helps your pecs look fabulous.

PUSH DOWN THE WALL. Stand about a foot away from the wall, and use your arm, chest, and shoulder muscles to push against the wall as hard as you can. See "Your Strength Training Guide at Home," page 246.

THROWING A MEDICINE BALL IS THE PERFECT MEDICINE FOR BUILDING A LEAN AND TONED UPPER BODY. Tossing this weighty ball back and forth with a partner is an unconventional way to gain upper-body strength while having fun.

Legs

SIT ON THE IMAGINARY CHAIR. And while doing this, you can imagine the newly toned and shapely legs you will have. Do this with your back against the wall, as described in "Your Strength Training Guide at Home," page 249.

WHO SAID THE LOCUST COMES AROUND ONLY EVERY SEVEN-TEEN YEARS? This locust should come several times per week. This yoga pose that looks like a backward leg lift strengthens and tones the glutes. See "Your Strength Training Guide at Home," page 249.

LOUNGING AROUND? Lunge around instead. See "Your Strength Training Guide at Home," page 249.

DON'T LET YOUR REAR BE THE BUTT OF JOKES. Do a lateral lunge. See "Your Strength Training Guide at Home," page 250.

BUTT-TONING MOVES CAN SHAPE YOUR HIPS, TOO! As a matter of fact, all butt-toning exercises do this, as the buttocks are the largest posterior hip muscles. Love that! So try any of our glute exercises in "Your Strength Training Guide at Home."

DO IT ON ALL FOURS! First, get your mind out of the gutter! Now, repeat the dog at the hydrant exercise three times with each leg. See "Your Strength Training Guide at Home," page 250.

STEP UP TO THE PLATE. No Stairmaster? Tone your butt on the staircase. This is a superior calorie-burning movement. You'll kill two birds with one stone—you reap both muscle-strengthening and cardiovascular benefits. See "Your Strength Training Guide at Home," page 249 and 250.

DON'T MAKE THIS LEGGY MISTAKE. Most males make the mistake of strengthening their upper bodies and overlooking their legs. Women make the mistake of focusing solely on the inner and outer thighs. Both are missing the boat when it comes to firing it up, as the leg muscles (quadriceps and hamstrings) are very large, and increasing lean muscle here can really help to speed up the metabolism.

Back

BEACH BALLS AREN'T ONLY FOR THE BEACH. See "Your Strength Training Guide at Home," page 246, to learn how to fire up all of your back muscles using a beach ball.

MONKEY BARS ONLY FOR KIDS? THAT'S MONKEY BUSINESS. Strengthen your upper body by using the strength of your back and arms to swing from one bar to another.

DON'T BE A PUSHOVER, TRY PULLING: EXERCISES THAT USE YOUR BACK. Most daily activities require us to use the "pushing" motion rather than the "pulling" motion. This causes our backs to be less muscular than our fronts. This muscular imbalance results in poor posture with shoulders that are rounded forward. A strong back pulls your shoulders back, making you have good posture and a cool, confident look. Not to mention pulling up breasts that may be lower than they used to be.

Your Strength Training Guide at Home

You don't need to perform every exercise. Just choose a couple of exercises for each muscle group for each exercise session. Next time you exercise that same muscle group, try a different exercise.

Most of these "at home" exercises can also be performed at the gym. However, we recommend hiring a personal trainer for at least your initial gym visit, so that he or she can help to familiarize you with all of the equipment and the proper way to use it. (Using the equipment properly is extremely important for preventing injuries and maximizing your workout.) Please note: We mention only the major muscle group(s) involved in each exercise. However, most exercises involve many smaller muscle groups as well.

Push-up (chest, shoulders, back)

Place hands on floor shoulder width apart. Place your feet on floor behind you so that your body is straight. Bend your elbows and lower your chest to the floor, then push up. (For an easier version, bend your knees and support your body weight with your hands and knees rather than with your hands and toes.) Be sure that your head is aligned with your body and is not sagging.

First set a goal of 10 push-ups, modified or classic. Work up to 3 sets every other day. After that, increase quantity of push-ups per set. The next step is to alternate the push-up with the bench press using a barbell, dumbbells, or a machine.

Wall push-down (chest)

Place your hands against a wall shoulder width apart. Stand about a foot away from the wall and push as hard as you can, as if you were going to knock the wall down. Hold for 30 seconds.

Repeat 3 times

Pretend you're Superman (lower back)

Lie flat on your stomach with your arms extended above your head. Lift your right arm and left leg as high as you can and hold for 10 seconds. Repeat with left arm and right leg.

3 sets of 10 reps on each side

Squeeze the beach ball (back)

Grab a beach ball and squish the ball into your chest as hard as you can. Hold for 30 seconds.

Repeat 3 times

Swing from the monkey bars (arms, back)

Hanging from the monkey bars, use your arms to "walk" from one bar to the next. Swing from bar to bar for 30 seconds.

Repeat 3 times

Bungee tubing for shoulders (see tip on using bungee tubing/cords on page 257)

Stand on one end of the cord. Hold the other end in your hand. Press your arm that is holding the bungee cord over your head. Keep your body still and lower your elbow so that your elbow is parallel with your shoulder. You should still feel some tension in the cord. Press your arm up straight so it is above your head.

3 sets of 12 reps per arm

Shoulder press

Pick up 2 hand weights and stand with your feet shoulder width apart. With your palms facing forward, and your hands up by your shoulders, raise your arms all the way while keeping your back straight and your stomach muscles tight. Slowly lower until your elbows form a 90-degree angle.

3 sets of 12 reps

Biceps curls

Pick up 2 hand weights. Stand up straight with your body aligned, head facing forward. With arms by your sides, palms facing forward, *slowly* curl your forearms up toward your shoulders by bending your elbows. Release slowly. Keep your wrists straight and be sure your body is still.

3 sets of 12 reps

Bungee tubing for biceps

Step on one end of the cord. Hold the other end in your hand, while standing up straight with your body aligned, head facing forward. Be sure that when your arm is down by your side there is some tension in the tubing. With your palm facing forward, slowly curl your arm up toward your shoulder by bending your elbow. Keep your wrist straight and your back straight and do not sway. Bend only your elbow.

3 sets of 12 reps for each arm

Dumbbell kick back (triceps)

Bend at the waist so your torso is about 45 degrees from upright. Hold a weight in each hand and position your upper arms parallel to the floor. Extend your lower arms straight backward. Slowly return to the start position.

3 sets of 12 reps

Triceps press

Hold a hand weight and lift your arm up above your head. Keeping your upper arm directly beside your head, and your elbow steady, bend your arm at the elbow until the weight almost touches your upper back. Slowly straighten your arm.

3 sets of 12 reps for each arm. As you get stronger, increase the weights.

Bungee tubing for triceps

Step on one end of the tubing and pull the other handle up behind your head. Bring your elbow up close to your ear and, with your arm bent behind you, extend your arm up until it is straight. You may hold your elbow close to your head with your other hand. Slowly lower back to the starting position.

12 reps for each arm; eventually, work your way up to 3 sets.

Posture pose (abs)

Keep your shoulders back and your abs tight and contracted. Stand up straight with your head facing forward.

Practice perfect posture all day long

Plank (abs)

Start on your knees and place your forearms on the ground with your fists together. Straighten your legs so that you are supporting your body weight with your forearms and toes. Keep your back flat and flex your stomach muscles, using them to prevent your body from sagging in the middle. Hold the position for as long as you can.

3 reps

Crunch (abs)

Lie on your back with your knees comfortably bent. Gently press your back into the floor and cross your hands across your chest. Holding your pelvis still, lift your shoulder blades off the floor, then lower them back down until your shoulders slightly brush the floor. Feel the tension from the top to the bottom of the abs. It is not necessary to lift high. Focus on the small contraction—a few inches is all you will need to lift.

3 sets of 20 reps

Reverse crunch (lower abs)

Lie on your back, your hands on the floor by your sides, and your knees bent and lifted off the floor (thighs should align over hips). Contract your abs and slowly roll your knees in toward your chin; lower to starting position. Don't use momentum to move knees. Your knees don't need to move more than an inch; just be sure it is your abs that are moving them.

3 sets of 15 reps

Locust (glutes)

Lie flat on your stomach with your arms at your sides (palms up and elbows tucked under your torso). Keeping both legs straight, lift one leg as high as it will go. Hold 10 seconds, then lower. (This looks like a backward leg lift). Repeat with other leg. Then raise both at same time, trying to raise thighs off floor.

Repeat 3 times

Frontal lunge (legs, butt)

Stand with feet shoulder width apart, abs tight, hands on hips. Lunge forward with one leg so that your thigh is parallel to the floor. Make sure your knee does not go farther forward than your toe. (Your shin should form a 90-degree angle with floor. Return to start.

3 sets of 12 reps per leg

Step-ups (or curb-ups) (legs, butt)

Step-ups: Climb a flight of stairs one at a time. Walk down slowly. Do this for 3 minutes. Then take two stairs at a time, and walk down slowly, one stair at a time. Then, if you can, take three stairs at a time, and walk down slowly, one stair at a time. Concentrate on squeezing your rear end to get the most tightening results.

Curb-ups: Step up on the curb with your right foot, then step up with your left foot. Step down with your right, then your left.

1 set of 15 beginning with right foot; 1 set of 15 beginning with left foot

Imaginary chair (legs)

Stand against a wall and use it as the back of your imaginary chair. Stand with legs about 1 to $1\frac{1}{2}$ feet away from the wall. Bend your legs until the tops of your thighs are parallel with the floor. Make sure that no more than a 90-degree angle is formed by the lower leg and thigh. Keep your back straight and your weight squarely over your heels. Try to hold for 30 seconds.

Repeat 3 times

Dog at hydrant (glutes, hamstrings, outer thighs)

Kneel with your hands, knees, and toes touching the ground. Keep your leg bent as you raise it toward the sky. Stop when the top of your leg is parallel with the floor. Hold for 2 seconds. Return to start position.

3 sets of 12 reps per leg

Lateral lunge (legs, glutes)

Stand with legs together. With your left leg, take a long step to the left and squat so that your thighs are parallel to the floor. Be sure that your knees are not in front of your toes. Return to start position.

3 sets of 12 reps per leg

Walking stairs (hamstrings, quadriceps)

Walk and climb stairs as part of your daily activities. Concentrate on contracting your glutes as you walk up the steps.

Work your way up to 20–30 minutes a day at a pace that simulates how you walk when late for an appointment.

Side shuffle (inner and outer thighs)

Shuffle to one side for 20 steps, than switch to the other side.

3 sets in each direction

Raise on tiptoes (calf)

Raise yourself up and down on your toes. Do this whenever you are standing around (e.g., brushing your teeth, waiting for the bus, at a crosswalk).

3 sets of 20 reps

Some of the following exercises can be performed at your home. You do not need to perform every exercise. Just pick one or two exercises for each muscle group for each exercise session. Next time you exercise that same muscle group, try a different exercise.

Your Strength Training Guide at the Gym

Just as with our "at home" exercises, we recommend hiring a personal trainer to help familiarize you with the equipment and the proper way to use it.

Free weight bench press (chest)

Lie on your back with your eyes directly under the supported bar. Place your feet on the bench so that your spine remains neutral (the way it is when in its natural upright position). Place your hands slightly wider than shoulder width apart. Lift the bar off its support and lower to the nipple line. Hold for 2 seconds and then extend your elbows and press the bar over the shoulders without locking the elbows. Pause. Note: Do not attempt this exercise unless you have a spotter who knows what he or she is doing.

3 sets of 12 reps

Pec deck (Chest)

Place your arms on the pads of the machine, with your elbows slightly below the level of your shoulders. Contract your abdominals to stabilize your body as you squeeze both pads together in front of your chest. Pause, then return to the starting position.

3 sets of 12 reps

Dumbbell flye (chest)

Lie faceup on a flat bench with your knees bent and feet placed on the edge of the bench. Hold one dumbbell in each hand, with your palms facing one another. Keeping your back flat on the bench, extend your arms directly above your chest with the dumbbells lightly touching. Do not straighten your arms completely. Slowly lower the dumbbells outward in an arc-like movement, until your arms are at shoulder level or slightly below. Pause, then use the same arc-like movement to return to starting position. (Picture yourself hugging a big beach ball.)

3 sets of 12 reps

Pull-up (back)

Grasp the bar with your hands shoulder width apart. Pull your body up until your chin is over the bar. Pause briefly. Then lower your body to the starting position. If you can't complete one pull-up, keep practicing. Pull yourself as high as you can go, even if it is only ¹/₂ inch, and pause briefly. Or if your gym has an assisted pull-up machine, use that to support some of your weight as you pull up.

3 sets of 12 reps

Lat pull-down (back)

Face the weight stack and sit, with your feet flat on the floor and your knees bent under the thigh pad. Grasp the bar slightly wider than shoulder width apart and with your palms facing the weight stack. Keeping your abdomen contracted, lean back 30 degrees from your hips. Squeeze your back muscles together as you pull the bar toward your chest. Pause, then return to extended position.

3 sets of 12 reps

Scapular adduction (shoulders)

Adjust the seat so that you are pulling at a height that is even with your shoulders while you are sitting. Place your feet flat on the floor, contract your abdomen, and grip the handles with your palms facing the ground. Keeping your arms straight (do not bend them at all during the exercise), squeeze your shoulder blades together. (You will actually move your arms only 4–6 inches.) Hold for several seconds and then release.

3 sets of 12 reps

Free weight one arm bent over dumbbell row (back)

Rest right hand, right knee, and lower right leg on a bench. Hold a dumbbell in your left hand and keep your spine neutral. Slightly bend your left knee and bend your hip at a 90-degree angle. Extend the left arm toward the floor and pull the dumbbell straight up toward your midback, keeping your elbow close to your side. Pause, then extend your arm to the starting position. Do not droop your shoulder or twist your back.

3 sets of 12 reps with each arm

Lateral shoulder raise

Stand with your back straight, feet approximately shoulder width apart, knees slightly bent, and abdominal muscles contracted. Hold a dumbbell in each hand. Extend arms down at sides and slightly bend elbows. Raise the dumbbells in a straight line out to your sides (palms facing floor) until your arms reach shoulder height. Pause and then slowly lower to starting position.

3 sets of 12 reps

Shoulder dumbbell press

Sit on an upright bench with a dumbbell in each hand. Contract your abs and put your arms at your sides, then raise the dumbbells over your head until they lightly touch. Pause, then slowly come back down to where both elbows are at a right angle. Avoid swinging your back, and relax your neck.

3 sets of 12 reps

Free weight seated incline biceps curl

Lie back on an incline bench, holding a dumbbell in each hand with an under-hand grip. Your arms should hang straight down with the palms forward. Curl both dumbbells up to shoulder height. Then lower them to full extension.

3 sets of 12 reps

Machine biceps curl

Adjust your arms so that the back of your arms rest comfortably on the pad. Make sure to keep your arms resting against the pad at all times. Relax your elbows, keep your wrists neutral, and grasp the bar with your hands shoulder width apart. While contracting your biceps, raise the bar to the top position. Slowly lower the bar to the start position (do not hyperextend your arms).

3 sets of 12 reps

Lying French press (triceps)

Lie faceup on the bench. Bend your knees and place your feet on the end of the bench. Press your lower back against the bench. Using both hands, hold a weighted bar overhead and keep your hands close together (about 6 inches apart). Keep your upper arms stationary and parallel to each other, and bend your forearms back and lower the weight behind and close to your head. Your elbows will remain pointing up. Pause, then slowly press the weight up over your head until your arms are fully extended and your hands are directly over your head. (Do not do this exercise without a spotter.)

3 sets of 12 reps

Triceps kickback

Place your right knee on the end of a bench. Holding a dumbbell in your left hand, lean forward and place your right hand on the other end of the bench for support. Keep your spine in a neutral position and contract your abdominals. Keeping your elbows relaxed and your left foot on the floor, extend your left elbow behind you until your arm is parallel to the floor and your palm is facing your torso. As you reach the top of the motion, really contract your triceps. Slowly return to the start position by bending your elbow to form a 90-degree angle with your triceps (your triceps should still be parallel to the floor).

3 sets of 12 reps for each arm

Crunch (abs)

Lie on your back on the floor with your knees comfortably bent. Gently press your back into the floor and cross your hands across your chest. Holding your pelvis still, lift your shoulder blades off the floor, then lower them back down until they slightly brush the floor. Feel the tension from the top to the bottom of the abs. It is not necessary to lift high. Focus on the small contraction—a few inches is all you will need to lift.

3 sets of 20 reps

Reverse crunch (lower abs)

Lie on your back, your hands on the floor by your sides and your knees bent and lifted off the floor (thighs should align over hips). Contract your abs and slowly roll your knees in toward your chin; lower to starting position. Don't use momentum to move knees. Your knees don't need to move more than an inch; just be sure it is your abs that are moving them.

3 sets of 15 reps

Rotation trunk curl (abdominal obliques)

Lie on your back with your knees bent and your feet a comfortable distance from your buttocks. Cross your left ankle over your right knee. Then place your hands at the sides of your head with your elbows out (do not clasp your hands). Rotate up and contract your abs, while keeping your head, neck, and shoulder blades in alignment. Cross your right shoulder (not elbow) over to your left knee. Pause at the top of the motion and then slowly return to the start position.

3 sets of 25 reps on each side; gradually increase to 50 reps

Pretend you're Superman (lower back)

Lie flat on your stomach with your arms extended above your head. Lift your right arm and left leg as high as you can and hold for 10 seconds. Repeat with left arm and right leg.

3 sets of 10 reps on each side

Horizontal leg press (buttocks, quadriceps, hamstrings)

Sit on the leg press machine with your feet shoulder width apart. Hold the handles. Contract your abdominals. Keeping your knees over your ankles and your entire foot in contact with the footplate, bend your knees to a 90-degree angle. Without locking your knees, straighten your legs. Slowly return to the start position.

3 sets of 12 reps

Leg extension (quadriceps)

Sit on the machine and hook your feet behind the pad. Adjust the machine so that it is comfortable and the leg extension arm is right below your shinbone. Slowly contract quadriceps and straighten legs. Pause, then slowly lower until you are at about a 30% angle of your start position (this will put less strain on your knees than returning all the way to the start position. When your legs are at the start position, they form a 90-degree angle). Pause.

3 sets of 12 reps

Leg curl (hamstrings)

Lie facedown on the machine, with your body against the bench pad. Make sure that the backs of your ankles are against the pads and your knees are in line with the rotating cam of the machine. Hold on to the handgrips and contract your hamstrings, slowly curling your legs up. Do not allow your hips to come up off the bench as your legs curl up. Pause at the top, then slowly lower back down to the start position.

3 sets of 12 reps

Hip adductor (inner thighs)

Sit with your back pressed into the machine and your hands gripping the handles. Press your feet and legs against the foam pads, contract your inner thigh muscles, and slowly and smoothly bring your legs together. Pause, then slowly return to starting position. Keep your legs and back in contact with the machine at all times.

3 sets of 12 reps

Hip abductor (outer thighs)

Sit with your back pressed into the machine and your hands gripping the handles. Press your feet and legs against the foam pads, contract your outer thigh muscles, and slowly and smoothly press your legs out. Pause, then slowly return to the starting position. Keep your legs and back in contact with the machine at all times.

3 sets of 12 reps

Standing heel raise (calves)

Center your shoulders on the pads of the machine and stand on the footplate of the calf machine. Contract your calves and slowly rise up on your toes. Pause briefly and lower your heels until they are fully extended. (If you don't have a calf machine, simply perform the same movement on the edge of a bottom step, while lightly holding on to the railing for stability.)

3 sets of 12 reps

TIPS

LIFTING WEIGHTS BEFORE CARDIO? ONLY IF YOU LIKE THE CARDIO BETTER. Starting your routine with the kind of exercise you like less makes it more likely that you will complete both cardio and the weights. On the other hand, if you leave what you like less for last, it is more likely to get left out. Just be sure to warm up for five minutes before whichever you choose to do.

DO IT MILITARY STYLE. Push-ups, squats, lunges—no excuses. You can do these muscle-strengthening exercises at home.

TUSHY TONERS AND TIGHTENERS—YOU CAN DO THESE ANY-WHERE. Just squeeze and tighten your tushy muscles. Do these at the desk, in the car, at the movies, and on the bus and you're sure to have a rear end that can crush.

IN A TIME CRUNCH? Focus on lifting weights with your back, chest, abs, or legs. Working these four large muscle groups rather than just the smaller ones (like the biceps and triceps) guarantees that more metabolism-revving muscles are built.

SHOCK YOUR MUSCLES TO BUILD EVEN MORE. Mix it up. Change your weight-lifting routine around. Switch among strength-training machines, dumbbells, and our out-of-the gym strength-training tips.

WALKING WITH HAND WEIGHTS? BETTER NOT. Your chance of injury is too high. You may strain your neck, back, and shoulders, and you may throw off your body alignment. Injuries can prevent you from exercising, and that will really slow your metabolism.

WHEN YOU LOWER, GO SLOWER. When you lower the weight after lifting it, do so very slowly. This lowering of the weight is called the eccentric phase of the lift, and when you do it slowly, it challenges the muscle even more, causing a longer rebuilding process and a longer post-metabolic boost.

Biceps, Triceps, and Shoulders

CAN IT! Don't belong to a gym? Don't have weights at home? No excuses. Pick up two canned foods of equal weights and begin.

BUNGEE CORDS FOR BUNGEE JUMPING? NOT THIS TIME. The only plunge you'll take is into a new, toned body. (You can purchase these inexpensive cords, also called tubes, at sporting goods stores, or even on-line, for your home gym.) Try bungee tubing for shoulders, biceps, and triceps. See "Your Strength Training Guide at Home," pages 246 to 248.

Legs: Smaller Muscle Groups

SHUFFLEBOARD, ANYONE? Actually, just do the side shuffle (similar to a gallop, but sideways) to one side for twenty steps, then switch to the other side. Do three sets. You'll really tone your inner and outer thighs. See "Your Strength Training Guide at Home," page 250.

BE ON YOUR TOES. At least sometimes. Walking around on your toes is a surefire way to build muscle tone and shape your calves and lower legs. Bonus: Your ankles will look smaller and your legs will look shapelier.

PUT A THICK PILLOW BETWEEN YOUR KNEES; PRESS YOUR LEGS TOGETHER AND SQUEEZE. These are so easy that you can do them on the couch while watching TV! Squeeze your legs together as hard as you can and hold for five seconds. Do this twelve times, then repeat twice. You'll feel a burn in your inner thighs. (You can also use a rolled-up bath towel.)

TWELVE

Sample Daily Menus for Levels 12, 14, and 16

We designed these menus to help you fire up your metabolism. You can use these menus any way you choose: You may want to follow them exactly for fourteen days to get the hang of eating the right foods at the right times. Or, if you feel as though you don't need to follow the menus, you can simply use them as a guide.

We provide menus for levels 12, 14, and 16. If you are a different level, simply add or subtract the appropriate servings so that the menu fits your level (as determined in Chapter 3, page 63).

Whenever you are hungry, fill up on vegetables (with the exception of potatoes, peas, and corn). Our vegetable portions are minimum requirements—feel free to have more. Also, you can season any vegetable at any meal with "I Can't Believe It's Not Butter" spray (not in the tub), or you can use any of the seasoning suggestions on page 67. Just be sure not to add any fat.

Habitual breakfast skippers: There is a special breakfast for you each day. Your breakfast portions will gradually increase so that your body isn't overwhelmed. Remember, your body is not accustomed to eating breakfast and is in a "conservation" mode, moving in slow gear. A normal-size breakfast is too much; your body will store some food as fat. Days 1 to 10 reflect Breakfast Banishers Cycle 1 options, and days 11 to 14 reflect Cycle 2 options, as every ten days portion sizes are increased.

Morning exercisers: Try to allow ½ to 1 hour for digestion before you exercise. If you cannot exercise with food in your stomach, eat breakfast immediately following your workout.

NOTE: If your level is level 12, be aware that your fat portions are very limited. Protein foods are used to extend carbohydrates' metabolic boost. (Your body does not burn very many calories, and if you ate more fat, the size of your meals would have to be extremely small.)

 # Day 1, Level 12

AFTER SLEEPING EIGHT FULL HOURS:

upon awakening	16 ounces of water
Breakfast: within 1 hour of awakening	½ cup Raisin Bran (Kellogg's or Post) (fits into your hand) ¾ cup skim or 1% milk (¾ size of your fist) **1 "always" carbohydrate, 1 "thumbs-up" protein**
Breakfast skippers:	¾ cup Raisin Bran, dry (Breakfast Banishers Cycle 1)
Midmorning snack: within 2½–3 hours after breakfast	4 ounces nonfat, light yogurt (like Dannon Light 'N Fit) (use toward protein servings) ¼ cup low-fat, no-sugar-added granola (sprinkled in yogurt) 16 ounces of water (sip throughout the morning) **1 "always" carbohydrate, ½ "thumbs-up" protein**

Lunch: 2–3 hours after midmorning snack	Mexican chicken wrap:
	   1 small whole wheat wrap (no bigger than the size of your stretched-out hand)
	   2 ounces chicken breast (not fried), cooked with cooking spray (like Pam) and low-sodium taco seasoning
	   ½ cup bell pepper, cooked
	   ¼ cup onion, cooked

$^1/_2$ cup squash, cooked

$^1/_2$ ounce (2 tablespoons) nonfat or low-fat cheese

1 cup cubed cantaloupe

8 ounces of water

**1 "always" carbohydrate, 1 fruit,
1$^1/_2$ "thumbs-up" proteins, 2$^1/_2$ vegetables**

Midafternoon snack
within 3–4 hours
after lunch

Red and green bell pepper strips (the more, the better)

1$^1/_2$ flat tablespoons hummus

8 ounces of water

$^1/_2$ vegetable, $^1/_2$ "friendly" fat

At the office,
about 20 minutes
before going out
to dinner with
coworkers

1 cup decaf or herb tea

Dinner at
seafood restaurant:
within 4 hours of
midafternoon snack

Large (about 2 cups) mixed green dinner salad with cherry
tomatoes, carrots, and balsamic vinegar (not vinaigrette)

4 ounces grilled swordfish steak (If more than 4 ounces,
share the rest with a friend, or save for tomorrow's lunch.)

1 cup cooked brown rice

1 cup steamed carrots, zucchini, and yellow squash

16 ounces of water

**2 "always" carbohydrates, 4 vegetables,
2 "thumbs-up" proteins**

After-dinner snack:
at least 1 hour
before bed

$^1/_2$ cup strawberries

1 fruit

Before bed   1 cup decaf or herb tea

**TODAY'S TOTALS: 1,240 calories; 5 carbohydrates, 5 proteins,
$^1/_2$ fat, 2 fruits, 7+ vegetables**

Day 2, Level 12

AFTER SLEEPING A FULL EIGHT HOURS:

Upon awakening	16 ounces of water
Breakfast: within 1 hour of awakening	Open-faced egg and cheese muffin: ½ whole wheat English muffin 2 scrambled egg whites 2 tablespoons shredded nonfat or low-fat cheese **1 "always" carbohydrate, 1 "thumbs-up" protein**
Breakfast skippers:	¼ whole wheat English muffin (can add I Can't Believe It's Not Butter spray) (Breakfast Banishers Cycle 1)
Midmorning snack: within 2½–3 hours after breakfast	¼ cup dried apricots (about 4–5 pieces) 1 tablespoon peanuts (prepackage the dried fruit and nuts in a Ziploc bag so that you can have it on the go) 16 ounces of water (sip throughout the morning) **1 fruit, ½ "friendly" fat**
Lunch: 2–3 hours after midmorning snack	2 cups Health Valley Italian Minestrone soup Spinach salad: 2 cups spinach ½ cup chopped tomatoes Seasoned rice vinegar or balsamic vinegar 8 ounces of water **1 "always" carbohydrate, 1 "thumbs-up" protein, 3 vegetables**
Midafternoon snack: within 3–4 hours after lunch	½ small (3" diameter, size of hockey puck) whole wheat bagel, topped with: ⅓ cup low-fat or ½ cup nonfat ricotta cheese and Sprinkle of fresh chives 8 ounces of water **1 "always" carbohydrate, 1 "thumbs-up" protein**

At the office, about 20 minutes before going home to make dinner	1 cup decaf or herb tea

Dinner: within 4 hours of midafternoon snack	4 ounces barbecued chicken breast 1 ear corn on the cob ½ cup steamed broccoli (topped with I Can't Believe It's Not Butter spray) ½ cup steamed cauliflower (topped with I Can't Believe It's Not Butter spray) 16 ounces of water **1 "always" carbohydrate, 2 vegetables, 2 "thumbs-up" proteins**

After-dinner snack: at least 1 hour before bed	1 cup nonfat, light yogurt (can count as protein or carbohydrate) 1 cup strawberries **1 "always" carbohydrate, 1 fruit**

Before bed	1 cup decaf or herb tea

TODAY'S TOTALS: 1,184 calories; 5 carbohydrates, 5 proteins, ½ fat, 2 fruits, 5+ vegetables

Day 3, Level 12

AFTER SLEEPING A FULL EIGHT HOURS:

Upon awakening	16 ounces of water
Breakfast: within 1 hour of awakening	2 slices reduced-calorie, high-fiber whole wheat toast, topped with: ½ cup nonfat ricotta cheese and ¼ cup crushed pineapple, drained **1 "always" carbohydrate, 1 "thumbs-up" protein, ½ fruit**
Breakfast skippers:	1 slice reduced-calorie, high-fiber whole wheat toast (with I Can't Believe It's Not Butter spray) (Breakfast Banishers Cycle 1)
Midmorning snack: within 2½–3 hours after breakfast	1 cup Cheerios 1 tablespoon mixed nuts (mix with Cheerios in a Ziploc bag so you can take it with you on the go) 16 ounces of water (sip throughout the morning) **1 "always" carbohydrate, ½ "friendly" fat**
Lunch: 2–3 hours after midmorning snack	Veggie Melt: ½ large whole wheat pita pocket ¾ ounce low-fat cheese or 1 ounce nonfat cheese 3 tomato slices 3 cucumber slices ¼ cup alfalfa sprouts 1½ tablespoons nonfat Italian dressing 10 baby carrots 8 ounces of water **1 "always" carbohydrate, 1 "thumbs-up" protein, 2 vegetables**

Midafternoon snack: within 3–4 hours after lunch	$^1/_8$ cantaloupe or honeydew melon 1 cup nonfat, light vanilla yogurt (put in melon) 8 ounces of water **1 fruit, 1 "thumbs-up" protein**
At the office, about 20 minutes before going home to make dinner	1 cup decaf or herb tea

Dinner: within 4 hours of midafternoon snack	Spaghetti with meat and vegetable sauce:
	    1 cup whole wheat pasta
	    2 ounces extra-lean ground beef (size of your
	      3 middle fingers)
	    $^1/_2$ cup each sliced bell peppers, squash, mushrooms,
	      and tomato sauce (look for sauces that have
	      50 calories or less in $^1/_2$ cup)
	    $^1/_2$ cup grilled eggplant (about four $^1/_2$" thick slices)
	    16 ounces of water
	
	 2 "always" carbohydrates, 3 vegetables,
	 1 "thumbs-up" protein

After-dinner snack: at least 1 hour before bed	1 Dannon Light 'N Fit nonfat strawberry yogurt (an "always" carbohydrate or a "thumbs-up" protein) 4 tablespoons blueberries **1 "thumbs-up" protein, $^1/_2$ fruit**
Before bed	1 cup decaf or herb tea

TODAY'S TOTALS: 1,223 calories; 5 carbohydrates, 5 proteins, $^1/_2$ fat, 2 fruits, 5+ vegetables

Day 4, Level 12

AFTER SLEEPING A FULL EIGHT HOURS:

Upon awakening   16 ounces of water

Breakfast: within 1 hour of awakening
½ cup cooked oatmeal with cinnamon (and Equal, if desired)
½ cup nonfat or low-fat cottage cheese (fits in the palm of your hand)

1 "always" carbohydrate, 1 "thumbs-up" protein

Breakfast skippers: ¼ cup oatmeal (Breakfast Banishers Cycle 1)

Midmorning snack: within 2½–3 hours after breakfast
½ apple
½ flat tablespoon peanut butter
16 ounces of water (sip throughout the morning)

½ fruit, ½ "friendly" fat

Lunch: 2–3 hours after midmorning snack
Turkey sandwich:
     2 slices reduced-calorie whole wheat bread
     2 ounces turkey breast
     2 leaves romaine lettuce
     3 slices tomato
     Mustard (optional)
8 baby carrots
½ cup cubed honeydew
8 ounces of water

1 "always" carbohydrate, 1 "thumbs-up" protein, ½ fruit, 2 vegetables

Midafternoon snack: within 3–4 hours after lunch	1 Veggie burger (such as Boca Burger Original or Veggie Burger) 1/2 whole wheat bun 1 slice tomato Ketchup (optional) 8 ounces of water **1 "thumbs-up" protein, 1 "always" carbohydrate**
At the office, about 20 minutes before going home to make dinner	1 cup decaf or herb tea

Dinner: within 4 hours of midafternoon snack	Shrimp or tofu stir-fry:
	   3 ounces shrimp or tofu
	   1/2 cup each steamed snow peas, carrots, and broccoli (can use frozen)
	   Cooking spray
	   3 tablespoons low-sodium soy sauce (1 tablespoon won't be enough)
	1 cup cooked brown rice
	16 ounces of water
	
	2 "always" carbohydrates, 3 vegetables, 1 1/2 "thumbs-up" proteins

After-dinner snack: at least 1 hour before bed	1 peach 1/2 cup nonfat, light vanilla yogurt **1 fruit, 1/2 "thumbs-up" protein**
Before bed	1 cup decaf or herb tea

TODAY'S TOTALS: 1,209 calories; 5 carbohydrates, 5 proteins, 2 fruits, 1/2 fat, 5+ vegetables

Day 5, Level 12

AFTER SLEEPING A FULL EIGHT HOURS:

Upon awakening	16 ounces of water

Breakfast: within 1 hour of awakening	French toast:
	    2 slices reduced-calorie, high-fiber whole wheat bread, dipped in:
	    2 egg whites and
	    ¹/₃ cup skim milk
	    Topped with 2 tablespoons sugar-free or 1 tablespoon light syrup, or 1 tablespoon low-sugar jelly
	
	1 "always" carbohydrate, 1 "thumbs-up" protein

Breakfast skippers:	¹/₂ slice whole wheat bread (Breakfast Banishers Cycle 1)
Midmorning snack: within 2¹/₂–3 hours after breakfast	³/₄ cup grapes 1 low-fat string cheese 16 ounces of water (sip throughout the morning) **1 fruit, 1 "thumbs-up" protein**

Lunch: 2–3 hours after midmorning snack	Tuna sandwich:
	    2 ounces tuna (canned in water)
	    ¹/₂ cup chopped onion and celery
	    1 tablespoon fat-free mayonnaise
	    2 slices tomato
	    2 romaine lettuce leaves
	    1 large whole wheat pita
	1¹/₂ cups veggie strips (bell peppers, broccoli florets, cauliflower florets)
	8 ounces of water
	
	2 "always" carbohydrates, 1 "thumbs-up" protein, 2¹/₂ vegetables

Midafternoon snack: within 3–4 hours after lunch	3 cups popcorn, popped (Healthy Choice or Pop Secret 94% Fat Free Butter) 1 tablespoon fat-free, fresh grated Parmesan cheese (sprinkled on popcorn) 8 ounces of water **1/2 "thumbs-up" protein, 1/2 "always" carbohydrate**
At the office, about 20 minutes before going home to make dinner	1 cup decaf or herb tea
Dinner: within 4 hours of midafternoon snack	3 ounces grilled salmon Grilled vegetable kabob (mushrooms, cherry tomatoes, yellow squash, zucchini), about 2 cups before being grilled 3/4 cup cooked brown rice or steamed quinoa 8 ounces of water **1 1/2 "thumbs-up" proteins, 1 1/2 "always" carbohydrates, 2 vegetables**
After-dinner snack: at least 1 hour before bed	1/4 cup raisins 1 tablespoon walnuts **1 fruit, 1/2 "friendly" fat**
Before bed	1 cup decaf or herb tea

TODAY'S TOTALS: 1,257 calories; 5 carbohydrates, 5 proteins, 2 fruits, 1/2 fat, 4 1/2+ vegetables

Day 6, Level 12

AFTER SLEEPING A FULL EIGHT HOURS:

Upon awakening	16 ounces of water
Breakfast: within 1 hour of awakening	2 tablespoons each pineapple chunks, mandarin oranges, chopped kiwi (totaling ½ cup) 1 cup nonfat plain yogurt or light, nonfat vanilla yogurt (mixed in fruit salad) 1 whole wheat pancake (4" diameter) 2 tablespoons sugar-free or 1 tablespoon light syrup, or 1 tablespoon low-sugar jelly **1 "always" carbohydrate, 1 fruit, 1 "thumbs-up" protein**
Breakfast skippers:	Just the fruit in the above breakfast (Breakfast Banishers Cycle 1)
Midmorning snack: within 2½–3 hours after breakfast	1 celery stalk ½ tablespoon peanut butter (put in celery canal) 16 ounces of water (sip throughout the morning) **½ vegetable, ½ "friendly" fat**
Lunch: 2–3 hours after midmorning snack	English muffin pizza: 　1 whole wheat English muffin 　½ cup tomato sauce 　½ cup sliced mushrooms 　½ cup chopped bell peppers 　1½ ounces nonfat cheese (2¼ pointer fingers) 8 ounces of water **2 "always" carbohydrates, 1½ "thumbs-up" proteins, 3 vegetables**

Midafternoon snack: within 3–4 hours after lunch	2 cups Health Valley Organic Lentil soup 8 ounces of water

1 "always" carbohydrate, 1 "thumbs-up" protein

At the office, about 20 minutes before going home to make dinner	1 cup decaf or herb tea

Dinner: within 4 hours of midafternoon snack	Orange chicken (recipe below): ¼ teaspoon olive oil ¼ small onion, chopped ½ cup sliced mushrooms Salt and pepper ⅛ cup water ⅛ teaspoon low-sodium soy sauce ½ teaspoon orange marmalade 3-ounce skinless chicken breast

1. Heat the olive oil in a large nonstick skillet and sauté the onion and mushrooms until tender.

2. Transfer to a bowl. Stir in salt and fresh ground pepper.

3. In a separate bowl, combine the water, soy sauce, and orange marmalade.

4. Place the chicken breast in the same skillet. Pour orange sauce over the chicken.

5. Bring to a boil, cover, and simmer for 20 minutes.

6. Add the mushroom mixture and simmer, uncovered, for 3 minutes.

1 cup steamed carrots, cauliflower, broccoli, and snow peas
1 whole wheat dinner roll
16 ounces of water

1 "always" carbohydrate, 1½ "thumbs-up" proteins, 2 vegetables

After-dinner snack: 1 baked apple topped with cinnamon
at least 1 hour
before bed

1 fruit

Before bed   1 cup decaf or herb tea

**TODAY'S TOTALS: 1,231 calories; 5 carbohydrates, 5 proteins,
2 fruits, ¹/₂ fat, 5¹/₂+ vegetables**

Day 7, Level 12

AFTER SLEEPING EIGHT FULL HOURS:

Upon awakening	16 ounces of water
Breakfast: within 1 hour of awakening	¼ cup Egg Beaters, scrambled ¼ cup each chopped peppers and onions, sautéed in cooking spray (mixed with eggs) 1 slice whole wheat toast (can use butter spray on top) 1 soy breakfast patty (like Morningstar Farms sausage patty) **1 "always" carbohydrate, 1½ "thumbs-up" proteins, 1 vegetable**
Breakfast skippers:	½ slice whole wheat toast (Breakfast Banishers Cycle 1)
Midmorning snack: within 2½–3 hours after breakfast	1 cup watermelon chunks 1 tablespoon pumpkin seeds 16 ounces of water (sip throughout the morning) **1 fruit, ½ "friendly" fat**
Lunch: 2–3 hours after midmorning snack	1 small (3 ounces) baked potato, topped with: ½ cup spiced chili beans and ¼ cup corn (canned okay, but not creamed) and ½ ounce nonfat American cheese 1 cup steamed broccoli 8 ounces of water **1½ "always" carbohydrates, 1½ "thumbs-up" proteins, 2 vegetables**
Midafternoon snack: within 3–4 hours after lunch	½ cup drained chickpeas, mixed with: ½ cup diced tomato and Juice of ½ lemon and pinch of salt and black pepper 8 ounces of water **1 "always" carbohydrate, 1 vegetable**

At the office,   1 cup decaf or herb tea
about 20 minutes
before going home
to make dinner

Dinner: Rosemary chicken (recipe below):
within 4 hours of   One 4-ounce chicken breast, with skin
midafternoon snack   Salt
Five-pepper blend
Fresh rosemary

1. In a heavy, nonstick skillet, place the chicken breast, skin side
   down. Sprinkle on salt and five-pepper blend.

2. Place a 3-inch branch of rosemary on the chicken.

3. Cover and cook over high heat, without turning, for 20–30 minutes.

4. Discard the chicken skin.

   $\frac{1}{2}$ cup each steamed yellow squash, zucchini, and
      carrots
   $\frac{3}{4}$ cup cooked brown rice
   16 ounces of water

   **1$\frac{1}{2}$ "always" carbohydrates, 2 "thumbs-up" proteins,
   3 vegetables**

After-dinner snack: $\frac{1}{2}$ pear, topped with:
at least 1 hour   1 tablespoon raisins and cinnamon
before bed

1 fruit

Before bed   1 cup decaf or herb tea

**TODAY'S TOTALS: 1,207 calories; 5 carbohydrates, 5 proteins,
$\frac{1}{2}$ fat, 2 fruits, 7+ vegetables**

Day 8, Level 12

AFTER SLEEPING A FULL EIGHT HOURS:

Upon awakening   16 ounces of water

Breakfast: 1 cup Fiber One cereal
within 1 hour of   ³/₄ cup skim milk
awakening

1 "always" carbohydrate, 1 "thumbs-up" protein

Breakfast skippers: ½ cup Fiber One cereal (Breakfast Banishers Cycle 1)

Midmorning   McDonald's Fruit and Yogurt Parfait (no granola)
snack: within   (count as both carbohydrate and protein)
2½–3 hours   16 ounces of water (sip throughout the morning)
after breakfast

1 "always" carbohydrate, 1 "thumbs-up" protein, 1 fruit

Lunch: 2–3 hours   Heat in microwave:
after midmorning   1 whole wheat English muffin, topped with:
snack   1½ tablespoons cranberry sauce (too little to count) and
    2 slices (2 ounces) fat-free honey-roasted turkey breast
    ½ cup grape tomatoes
    ½ cup cauliflower florets
    8 ounces of water

**2 "always" carbohydrates, 1 "thumbs-up" protein,
2 vegetables**

Midafternoon   1 cup carrot and celery strips
snack: within 3–4   ½ tablespoon cashew butter (for dipping)
hours after lunch   8 ounces of water

1 vegetable, ½ "friendly" fat

At the office, about 20 minutes before going home to make dinner	1 cup decaf or herb tea
Dinner: within 4 hours of midafternoon snack	Mexican fajita (recipe below):

Mexican fajita (recipe below):
- ¹/₂ tablespoon fat-free Italian dressing
- ¹/₂ tablespoon lemon or lime juice
- ¹/₄ medium onion, thinly sliced
- 1 small red or green pepper, cut into thick strips
- 4 ounces precut extra-lean beef (such as round steak) or skinless chicken breast
- Salsa (optional)
- One 6" whole wheat tortilla

1. *In a large, nonstick skillet, combine the Italian dressing and lemon or lime juice. Add the onion and cook over medium heat for 1¹/₂ minutes.*

2. *Add the pepper and cook, stirring, about 1 minute.*

3. *Add the meat and cook, stirring, for 1 minute.*

4. *Top with salsa.*

5. *Serve wrapped inside tortilla.*

¹/₂ cup steamed zucchini
16 ounces of water

1 "always" carbohydrate, 2 "thumbs-up" proteins, 2 vegetables

After-dinner snack: at least 1 hour before bed	¹/₂ cup fresh raspberries

1 fruit

Before bed	1 cup decaf or herb tea

TODAY'S TOTALS: 1,203 calories; 5 carbohydrates, 5 proteins, 2 fruits, ¹/₂ fat, 5+ vegetables

Day 9, Level 12

AFTER SLEEPING A FULL EIGHT HOURS:

Upon awakening   16 ounces of water

Breakfast: 1 whole-grain waffle (like Eggo Nutri-Grain Multigrain),
within 1 hour of   topped with:
awakening   ½ cup nonfat, light vanilla yogurt and
        2 tablespoons low-calorie, sugar-free syrup or
            1 tablespoon light syrup

1 "always" carbohydrate, ½ "thumbs-up" protein

Breakfast skippers: ½ waffle with 1 tablespoon low-calorie, sugar-free syrup
        (Breakfast Banishers Cycle 1)

Midmorning   Trail mix (make yourself by mixing peaches and raisins,
snack: within   and package in Ziploc baggie to eat on the run)
2½–3 hours   3 dried peach halves
after breakfast   1 teaspoon raisins
    2 hard-boiled egg whites
    16 ounces of water (sip throughout the morning)

1 fruit, ½ "thumbs-up" protein

Lunch: 2–3 hours   Grilled cheese pita sandwich (combine all ingredients in
after midmorning   pita and heat in microwave until cheese is melted)
snack   ½ whole wheat pita
        1 ounce nonfat cheese
        ¾ cup shredded romaine lettuce
        ¼ cup shredded carrots
        ½ apple, diced
        4 tablespoons nonfat Italian dressing
    1 cup celery and carrot sticks
    8 ounces of water

**1 "always" carbohydrate, 1 "thumbs-up" protein, ½ fruit,
2 vegetables**

Midafternoon snack: within 3–4 hours after lunch	2 Carr's Whole Wheat crackers covered with: ⅓ cup low-fat cottage cheese mixed with chives or onion dip 8 ounces of water

1 "always" carbohydrate, 1 "thumbs-up" protein

At the office, about 20 minutes before going home for dinner	1 cup decaf or herb tea

Dinner: within 4 hours of midafternoon snack	Order in Chinese: 1 cup brown rice 4 ounces steamed chicken or seafood At least 2 cups steamed vegetables (eggplant, broccoli, string beans, mushrooms, snow peas, water chestnuts) 2 tablespoons garlic sauce, drizzled on top (order sauce on the side) Low-sodium soy sauce 16 ounces of water

2 "always" carbohydrates, 2 "thumbs-up" proteins, ½ "friendly" fat, 4 vegetables

After-dinner snack: at least 1 hour before bed	¼ cup berries

½ fruit

Before bed	1 cup decaf or herb tea

TODAY'S TOTALS: 1,247 calories; 5 carbohydrates, 5 proteins, ½ fat, 2 fruits, 6+ vegetables

Day 10, Level 12

AFTER SLEEPING A FULL EIGHT HOURS:

Upon awakening   16 ounces of water

Breakfast: Yogurt parfait (recipe below):
within 1 hour of   1/2 cup sugar-free, nonfat vanilla yogurt
awakening   1/8 teaspoon ground cinnamon
        1/4 cup sliced strawberries
        1/8 cup blueberries
        1/8 cup raspberries
        1/4 cup low-fat granola without raisins

1. Combine the yogurt and cinnamon in a small bowl.

2. Combine the berries in another bowl.

3. Layer the fruit mixture, yogurt, and granola in a parfait glass.

**1 "sometimes" carbohydrate, 1/2 "thumbs-up" protein,
1 fruit**

Breakfast skippers: 1/2 cup (4 ounces) sugar-free, nonfat yogurt (Breakfast
        Banishers Cycle 1)

Midmorning   3 cups air-popped popcorn
snack: within   2 teaspoons grated Parmesan (mixed into popcorn)
2 1/2–3 hours   16 ounces of water (sip throughout the morning)
after breakfast

1 "always" carbohydrate, 1 "thumbs-up" protein

Lunch: 2–3 hours   Wendy's Mandarin Chicken Salad (use 1/3 of the Oriental
after midmorning   Sesame dressing, about 2 tablespoons; hold the noodles
snack   and almonds)
    8 ounces of water

**2 "thumbs-up" proteins, 1 fruit, 1/2 "friendly" fat,
1 1/2 vegetables**

Midafternoon snack: within 3–4 hours after lunch	½ small baked potato
	½ cup steamed broccoli (on potato)
	½ ounce nonfat cheddar cheese (on potato)
	8 ounces of water

½ "always" carbohydrate, ½ "thumbs-up" protein, 1 vegetable

| At the office, about 20 minutes before going home to make dinner | 1 cup decaf or herb tea |

Dinner: within 4 hours of midafternoon snack	Spicy egg burrito (recipe below):
	5 tablespoons nonfat egg substitute
	½ tablespoon diced mild green chilies
	2 tablespoons shredded nonfat cheddar cheese
	1 tablespoon fresh cilantro
	One 7" whole wheat tortilla
	1 tablespoon salsa
	1 tablespoon nonfat sour cream
	1 green onion (scallion), thinly sliced and divided

1. *Spray a nonstick skillet with cooking spray.*

2. *Add the egg substitute and chilies and cook, stirring, over medium heat until eggs are softly set, about 2 minutes.*

3. *Stir in the cheese and cilantro.*

4. *Continue cooking and folding until the eggs are cooked to desired doneness, about 1 minute.*

5. *Wrap the tortilla in a paper towel and microwave on high for about 10 seconds or until hot.*

6. *Place the eggs in the center of the tortilla. Roll up and face seam side down.*

7. *Top with salsa, sour cream, and green onion.*

1 cup steamed squash, broccoli, and cauliflower
16 ounces of water

**1 "always" carbohydrate, 1 "thumbs-up" protein,
2½ vegetables**

After-dinner snack: ½ whole wheat pita, heated and cut into triangles
at least 1 hour ¼ cup fat-free bean dip (count as carbohydrate)
before bed

1½ "always" carbohydrates

Before bed 1 cup decaf or herb tea

**TODAY'S TOTALS 1,194 calories; 5 carbohydrates (4 "always,"
1 "sometimes"), 5 proteins, ½ fat, 2 fruits, 5+ vegetables**

Day 11, Level 12

AFTER SLEEPING A FULL EIGHT HOURS:

Upon awakening	16 ounces of water
Breakfast: within 1 hour of awakening	½ cup nonfat or 1% cottage cheese, topped with: ⅓ cup warmed canned (in water or juice, not syrup) or fresh peaches 1 slice whole wheat bread

1 "always" carbohydrate, 1 "thumbs-up" protein, ¾ fruit

Breakfast skippers:	1 slice whole wheat bread (you can add I Can't Believe It's Not Butter spray) (Breakfast Banishers Cycle 2)

Midmorning snack: within 2½–3 hours after breakfast	3 Ry-Krisp crackers 1 slice (3 ounces) extra-thin-sliced deli turkey breast (like Hillshire Farms) 16 ounces of water (sip throughout the morning)

1 "always" carbohydrate, ½ "thumbs-up" protein

Lunch: 2–3 hours after midmorning snack	open-faced portobello mushroom burger:
	    1 large portobello mushroom cap, sautéed in olive oil cooking spray
	    ¾ ounce nonfat cheddar cheese
	    3 slices tomato
	    Onion, several slices
	    ½ whole-grain bun
	 Strawberry salad:
	    1 cup chopped romaine lettuce
	    ½ cup chopped strawberries
	    1 spray olive oil from spray bottle
	    Balsamic vinegar to taste
	    1 tablespoon slivered almonds (only if you do not use light mayo with midafternoon snack)
	 8 ounces of water

1 "always" carbohydrate, 3/4 "thumbs-up" protein, 1 fruit, 1/2 "friendly" fat (if you eat the almonds), 2 1/2 vegetables

Midafternoon snack: within 3–4 hours after lunch

1/2 Chicken McGrill sandwich (share other half with a friend), use only 1 tablespoon light mayo (better: Use ketchup or mustard on sandwich and add almonds to salad at lunch, as light mayo is a fat "foe")
8 ounces of water

1 "sometimes" carbohydrate, 1 "thumbs-up" protein, 1/2 vegetable

At the office, about 20 minutes before going home to make dinner

1 cup decaf or herb tea

Dinner: within 4 hours of midafternoon snack

Salmon and dill (recipe below):
1/4 cup plain nonfat yogurt
1/2 teaspoon fresh or 1/4 teaspoon dried dill
1/2 teaspoon lemon juice
Salt
3-ounce salmon fillet
1 cup steamed spinach

1. Preheat the oven to 350 degrees.

2. Whisk together the yogurt, dill, lemon juice, and salt.

3. Pour the mixture over the salmon fillet.

4. Bake for 10 minutes.

5. Serve over steamed spinach

2 small (together, not bigger than your fist) red-skin potatoes mashed with fat-free chicken broth
16 ounces of water

1 "always" carbohydrate, 1 3/4 "thumbs-up" proteins, 2 vegetables

After-dinner snack: $1/4$ cup cubed cantaloupe
     at least 1 hour
       before bed

               $1/4$ fruit

Before bed   1 cup decaf or herb tea

TODAY'S TOTALS: 1,192 calories; 5 carbohydrates (4 "always," 1 "sometimes"), 5 proteins, $1/2$ fat, 2 fruits, 5+ vegetables

Day 12, Level 12

AFTER SLEEPING A FULL EIGHT HOURS:

Upon awakening 16 ounces of water

Breakfast: Raisin French toast (recipe below):
within 1 hour of   ½ teaspoon vanilla extract
awakening   3 egg whites, or ½ cup fat-free egg substitute
                    1 slice whole wheat raisin bread (like Baker's)
                    2 tablespoons sugar-free or 1 tablespoon light syrup,
                        or 2 teaspoons low-sugar jelly

1. Mix the vanilla extract and egg whites.

2. Dip the bread in the egg mixture, coating both sides.

3. Cook in a preheated nonstick frying pan until both sides are light brown.

4. Top with syrup or jelly.

1 "always" carbohydrate, ³/₄ "thumbs-up" protein

Breakfast skippers: 1 slice whole wheat raisin bread (butter spray optional)
                     (Breakfast Banishers Cycle 2)

Midmorning   1 apple
snack: within   1 low-fat string cheese
2½–3 hours   16 ounces of water (sip throughout the morning)
after breakfast

1 fruit, 1 "thumbs-up" protein

Lunch: 2–3 hours 1 veggie frank (like Natural Touch Vege Frank)
after midmorning 1 tablespoon each ketchup and mustard for dipping
snack   (optional)
                  ½ cup baked beans (vegetarian, no pork, etc.)
                  1 cup onions and green and red bell peppers, sautéed in
                      cooking spray
                  8 ounces of water

1 "always" carbohydrate, 1¼ "thumbs-up" proteins, 2 vegetables

Midafternoon snack: within 3–4 hours after lunch

1 cup Health Valley Lentil and Carrot soup
8 ounces of water

½ "always" carbohydrate, ½ "thumbs-up" protein

At the office, about 20 minutes before going home to make dinner

1 cup decaf or herb tea

Dinner: within 4 hours of midafternoon snack

Beef stir-fry (recipe below):
  3 ounces extra-lean beef (such as flank steak), cut in strips
  1 teaspoon canola oil
  1 teaspoon fresh, minced ginger
  1 clove minced garlic
  ½ cup snow peas
  ¼ cup water chestnuts
  ½ cup bean sprouts
  ½ cup broccoli florets
  ½ cup chopped bell pepper
  1 tablespoon reduced-sodium soy sauce
  ½ teaspoon sugar
  1 cup cooked brown rice

1. Brown the beef in a nonstick skillet. Remove beef from skillet and put on plate.

2. Add canola oil to the skillet and sauté the ginger and garlic. Add the vegetables and cook until still crunchy.

3. Stir in the soy sauce and sugar.

4. Put the beef in the sauce, briefly, to rewarm.

5. Serve over brown rice.

16 ounces of water

2 "always" carbohydrates, 1½ "thumbs-up" proteins, ½ "friendly" fat, 4½ vegetables

After-dinner snack: ½ cup nonfat, light cherry yogurt (count as carbohydrate)
at least 1 hour ¾ cup cherries (stirred in yogurt)
before bed

½ "always" carbohydrate, 1 fruit

Before bed 1 cup decaf or herb tea

TODAY'S TOTALS: 1,268 calories; 5 carbohydrates, 5 proteins, 2 fruits, ½ fat, 6½+ vegetables

Day 13, Level 12

AFTER SLEEPING A FULL EIGHT HOURS:

Upon awakening	16 ounces of water

Breakfast: within 1 hour of awakening	Peachy smoothie
	In a blender, combine:
	   1 cup nonfat, light peach yogurt (count as
	      $^3/_4$ carbohydrate and $^1/_4$ protein)
	   $^1/_4$ cup frozen peaches
	   $^1/_4$ cup frozen raspberries
	   Several ice cubes

$^3/_4$ "always" carbohydrate, $^1/_4$ "thumbs-up" protein, 1 fruit

Breakfast skippers:	Blend $^1/_2$ cup yogurt, $^1/_4$ cup frozen berries, and ice cubes (Breakfast Banishers Cycle 2)
Midmorning snack: within $2^1/_2$–3 hours after breakfast	$^1/_2$ large banana, sliced, mixed into: $^1/_4$ cup nonfat sour cream 16 ounces of water (sip throughout the morning)

1 "thumbs-up" protein, 1 fruit

Lunch: 2–3 hours after midmorning snack	Crab-stuffed tomato (recipe below):
	   2 ounces canned crabmeat, drained
	   2 teaspoons fat-free mayonnaise
	   1 teaspoon fresh lemon juice
	   1 teaspoon fresh dill, stuffed
	   1 small tomato, cut in half, seeds and pulp scooped out

1. *Mix together the crabmeat, mayonnaise, lemon juice, and dill.*

2. *Stuff half of the mixture into each tomato half.*

      1 slice reduced-calorie whole wheat bread (with butter spray)

2 cups watercress and cucumber salad

2 tablespoons fat-free Italian dressing

8 ounces of water

½ "always" carbohydrate, 1 "thumbs-up" protein, 2½ vegetables

Midafternoon snack: within 3–4 hours after lunch

Barley and bean salad

Mix together:

  ½ cup cooked barley

  ½ cup chopped cucumber

  ½ cup chopped tomato

  1½ tablespoons red kidney beans

  1 teaspoon olive oil

  2 teaspoons red wine vinegar

  8 ounces of water

1 "always" carbohydrate, ⅓ "thumbs-up" protein, ½ "friendly" fat, 2 vegetables

At the office, about 20 minutes before going home to make dinner

1 cup decaf or herb tea

Dinner: within 4 hours of midafternoon snack

Crispy oven-fried fired-up chicken (recipe below):

  1 egg white, beaten

  Oregano, pepper, salt, minced onion, and garlic (to taste)

  ½ tablespoon flour

  3-ounce skinless chicken breast

  ½ cup Bran Flakes

1. Preheat the oven to 350 degrees.

2. Combine the egg white and spices.

3. Pat flour on both sides of the chicken breast so that it has a very light coating.

4. Dip the chicken breast in the egg white and spice mixture.

5. Dip the chicken breast in the Bran Flakes and coat on both sides.

6. Bake for 30–45 minutes.

> $^3/_4$ cup steamed asparagus
> $^1/_4$ cup steamed carrots
> 1 small (3 ounces, about 4" long) sweet potato, mashed
>   with 2 tablespoons orange juice
> 16 ounces of water
>
> **1$^3/_4$ "always" carbohydrates, 1$^3/_4$ "thumbs-up" proteins,
> 2 vegetables**

After-dinner snack: Root beer float
at least 1 hour $^1/_2$ cup nonfat frozen yogurt
before bed $^1/_2$ cup skim milk mixed with 1 diet cream soda

1 "rarely" carbohydrate, $^2/_3$ "thumbs-up" protein

Before bed   1 cup decaf or herb tea

**TODAY'S TOTALS: 1,211 calories; 5 carbohydrates (4 "always,"
1 "rarely"), 5 proteins, 2 fruits, $^1/_2$ fat, 6$^1/_2$+ vegetables**

Day 14, Level 12

AFTER SLEEPING A FULL EIGHT HOURS:

Upon awakening   16 ounces of water

Breakfast:
within 1 hour of
awakening

1 hard-boiled egg mashed with 1 tablespoon fat-free
     mayonnaise
½ whole wheat English muffin (spread egg salad on top)

1 "always" carbohydrate, 1 "thumbs-up" protein

Breakfast skippers:

½ whole wheat English muffin (butter spray optional)
     (Breakfast Banishers Cycle 2)

Midmorning
snack: within
2½–3 hours
after breakfast

1 slice Canadian bacon
1 slice whole wheat, reduced-calorie bread (with
     I Can't Believe It's Not Butter spray)
16 ounces of water (sip throughout the morning)

½ "always" carbohydrate, ½ "thumbs-up" protein

Lunch: 2–3 hours
after midmorning
snack

Tuna melt (recipe below):
     1 ounce tuna (canned in water)
     1 tablespoon chopped onion
     1 tablespoon chopped celery
     1 tablespoon nonfat mayonnaise (or mustard or vinegar)
     2 slices reduced-calorie whole wheat bread, or ½ large
         whole wheat pita
     ½ ounce nonfat cheese

1. Mix together the tuna, onion, celery, and mayonnaise.

2. Put the mixture on 1 slice of bread and top with the cheese.

3. Put under the broiler to melt the cheese.

4. Place the other slice of bread on top.

Tomato artichoke salad:
     2 cups torn romaine lettuce
     ½ cup cooked artichoke hearts, quartered

1 large plum tomato, sliced
1 tablespoon fat-free Italian dressing
8 ounces of water

1 "always" carbohydrate, 1 "thumbs-up" protein, 2½ vegetables

Midafternoon snack: within 3–4 hours after lunch	1½ kiwis, sliced 4 ounces nonfat, light vanilla yogurt (mix with fruit and cereal) 2 tablespoons Grape-Nuts cereal 8 ounces of water

½ "always" carbohydrate, ½ "thumbs-up" protein, 1 fruit

At the office, about 20 minutes before going out to dinner with coworkers	1 cup decaf or herb tea

Dinner at Japanese restaurant: within 4 hours of midafternoon snack	Appetizer of ⅓ cup edamame beans 1 avocado and cucumber roll (6 pieces), made with brown rice 1 tuna roll (6 pieces), made with brown rice Side salad, ginger dressing on the side (eaten with "fork-dipping" tactic) 16 ounces of water

2 "always" carbohydrates, 2 "thumbs-up" proteins, ¾ "friendly" fat, 2¼ vegetables

After-dinner snack: at least 1 hour before bed	½ mango

1 fruit

Before bed	1 cup decaf or herb tea

Today's totals: 1,257 calories; 5 carbohydrates, 5 proteins, 2 fruits, ¾ fat, 4¾+ vegetables

Day 1, Level 14

The same menu as Day 1, Level 12, except:

Midmorning snack   Have 6 ounces of yogurt with the granola.

1 "always" carbohydrate, ³/₄ "thumbs-up" protein

Midafternoon snack   Have 3 flat tablespoons of hummus with the bell pepper strips (the more the better).

1 vegetable, 1 fat

Dinner   Add 2 tablespoons slivered almonds to the salad.

2 "always" carbohydrates, 4 vegetables, 2 "thumbs-up" proteins, 1 fat

---

TODAY'S TOTALS: 1,407 calories; 5 carbohydrates, 5¼ proteins, 2 fats, 2 fruits, 7+ vegetables

Day 2, Level 14

The same menu as Day 2, Level 12, except:

Midmorning snack   Have 2 tablespoons peanuts with the apricots.

1 fruit, 1 "friendly" fat

Lunch   Add ¼ cup mashed avocado, ½ cup sliced bell peppers, and ½ cup sliced carrots to the spinach salad.

1 "always" carbohydrate, 1 "thumbs-up" protein, 1 "friendly" fat, 5 vegetables

---

TODAY'S TOTALS: 1,381 calories; 5 carbohydrates, 5 proteins, 2 fats, 2 fruits, 7+ vegetables

Day 3, Level 14

The same menu as Day 3, Level 12, except:

Midmorning snack   Have 2 tablespoons mixed nuts with the Cheerios.

1 "always" carbohydrate, 1 "friendly" fat

Midafternoon snack   Add 2 tablespoons sunflower seeds to the melon and yogurt.

1 fruit, 1 "thumbs-up" protein, 1 "friendly" fat

TODAY'S TOTALS: 1,377 calories; 5 carbohydrates, 5 proteins, 2 fats, 2 fruits, 5+ vegetables

Day 4, Level 14

The same menu as Day 4, Level 12, except:

Midmorning snack   Have 1 flat tablespoon peanut butter with the ½ apple.

½ fruit, 1 "friendly" fat

Dinner   Use 1 teaspoon sesame oil (instead of cooking spray) and add 1 tablespoon sesame seeds to the stir-fry.

2 "always" carbohydrates, 3 vegetables, 1½ "thumbs-up" proteins, 1 "friendly" fat

---

TODAY'S TOTALS: 1,343 calories; 5 carbohydrates, 5 proteins, 2 fruits, 2 fats, 5+ vegetables

Day 5, Level 14

The same menu as Day 5, Level 12, except:

Breakfast   Also top the French toast with 2 tablespoons pecan halves.

**1 "always" carbohydrate, 1 "thumbs-up" protein,
1 "friendly" fat**

After-dinner snack   Have 2 tablespoons walnuts with the raisins.

1 fruit, 1 "friendly" fat

**TODAY'S TOTALS: 1,368 calories; 5 carbohydrates, 5 proteins,
2 fruits, 2 fats, 4¹/₂+ vegetables**

Day 6, Level 14

The same menu as Day 6, Level 12, except:

Midmorning snack   Put 1 tablespoon peanut butter in the celery stalk.

1 "friendly fat," ¹/₂ vegetable

After-dinner snack   Put 2 tablespoons sliced pecans on top of the baked apple.

1 "friendly" fat, 1 fruit

**TODAY'S TOTALS: 1,382 calories; 5 carbohydrates, 5 proteins,
2 fruits, 2 fats, 5¹/₂+ vegetables**

Day 7, Level 14

The same menu as Day 7, Level 12, except:

Midmorning snack   Have 2 tablespoons pumpkin seeds with the watermelon.

1 fruit, 1 "friendly" fat

Midafternoon snack   Add 2 teaspoons olive oil to the chickpea salad.

1 "always" carbohydrate, 1 vegetable, 1 "friendly" fat

TODAY'S TOTALS: 1,375 calories; 5 carbohydrates, 5 proteins, 2 fats, 2 fruits, 7+ vegetables

Day 8, Level 14

The same menu as Day 8, Level 12, except:

Midafternoon snack   Have 1 tablespoon cashew butter for dipping the celery and carrot strips.

1 "friendly" fat, 1 vegetable

After-dinner snack   Add 2 tablespoons slivered almonds to the raspberries.

1 fruit, 1 "friendly" fat

TODAY'S TOTALS: 1,350 calories; 5 carbohydrates, 5 proteins, 2 fruits, 2 fats, 5+ vegetables

Day 9, Level 14

The same menu as Day 9, Level 12, except:

Breakfast   Add 2 tablespoons slivered pecans to the waffle topping.

1 "always" carbohydrate, ½ "thumbs-up" protein,
1 "friendly" fat

Dinner   Use 4 tablespoons garlic sauce.

2 "always" carbohydrates, 2 "thumbs-up" proteins,
1 "friendly" fat, 4 vegetables

TODAY'S TOTALS: 1,402 calories; 5 carbohydrates, 5 proteins,
2 fats, 2 fruits, 6+ vegetables

Day 10, Level 14

The same menu as Day 10, Level 12, except:

Lunch   Use the almond packet on the chicken salad (still hold
the noodles).

2 "thumbs-up" proteins, 1 fruit, 2 "friendly" fats,
1½ vegetables

TODAY'S TOTALS: 1,340 calories; 5 carbohydrates (4 "always,"
1 "sometimes"), 5 proteins, 2 fats, 2 fruits, 5+ vegetables

Day 11, Level 14

The same menu as Day 11, Level 12, except:

Lunch   Have 2 tablespoons slivered almonds on the strawberry salad.

1 "always" carbohydrate, ³/₄ "thumbs-up protein," 1 fruit, 1 "friendly" fat, 2¹/₂ vegetables

Midafternoon snack   Add 2 flat tablespoons of light mayo to Chicken McGrill sandwich (or use mustard or ketchup on the sandwich and add 4 tablespoons almonds to salad at lunch)

1 "sometimes" carbohydrate, 1 "thumbs-up" protein, 1 fat "foe," ¹/₂ vegetable

---

TODAY'S TOTALS: 1,348 calories; 5 carbohydrates (4 "always," 1 "sometimes"), 5 proteins, 2 fats (1 "friendly," 1 "foe"), 2 fruits, 5+ vegetables

Day 12, Level 14

The same menu as Day 12, Level 12, except:

Midmorning snack   Cut the apple in quarters and spread 1 flat tablespoon peanut butter on the apple pieces.

1 fruit, 1 "thumbs-up" protein, 1 "friendly" fat

After-dinner snack   Add 1 tablespoon sunflower seeds to the yogurt.

¹/₂ "always" carbohydrate, 1 fruit, ¹/₂ fat

TODAY'S TOTALS: 1,414 calories; 5 carbohydrates, 5 proteins, 2 fruits, 2 fats, and 6¹/₂+ vegetables

Day 13, Level 14

The same menu as Day 13, Level 12, except:

Midmorning snack   Add 2 tablespoons slivered almonds or another nut of your choice to the bananas and cream.

1 "thumbs-up" protein, 1 fruit, 1 "friendly" fat

Lunch   Add 1 ounce (about 4 small cubes) avocado to watercress and cucumber salad.

¹/₂ "always" carbohydrate, 1 "thumbs-up" protein, ¹/₂ "friendly" fat, 2¹/₂ vegetables

TODAY'S TOTALS: 1,358 calories; 5 carbohydrates (4 "always," 1 "rarely"), 5 proteins, 2 fruits, 2 fats, 6¹/₂+ vegetables

Day 14, Level 14

The same menu as Day 14, Level 12, except:

Midmorning snack   Have 1¹/₄ tablespoons peanut butter on the bread.

¹/₂ "always" carbohydrate, ¹/₂ "thumbs-up" protein, 1¹/₄ "friendly" fats

TODAY'S TOTALS: 1,399 calories; 5 carbohydrates, 5 proteins, 2 fruits, 2 fats, 4³/₄+ vegetables

Day 1, Level 16

The same menu as Day 1, Level 12, except:

Breakfast
Have 1 cup Raisin Bran and 1¼ cups milk.
2 "always" carbohydrates, 1½ "thumbs-up" proteins

Midmorning snack
Have 8 ounces of yogurt.
1 "always" carbohydrate, 1 "thumbs-up" protein

Lunch
Eat 3 ounces chicken breast in the wrap.
1 "always" carbohydrate, 1 fruit, 2 "thumbs-up" proteins, 2½ vegetables

Midafternoon snack
Have 3 flat tablespoons hummus.
½ vegetable, 1 "friendly" fat

Dinner
Add 2 tablespoons slivered almonds to the dinner salad.
1 "friendly" fat, 2 "always" carbohydrates, 4 vegetables, 2 "thumbs-up" proteins

TODAY'S TOTALS: 1,623 calories; 6 carbohydrates, 6½ proteins, 2 fats, 2 fruits, 7+ vegetables

Day 2, Level 16

The same menu as Day 2, Level 12, except:

Breakfast
Have 1 whole wheat English muffin, 4 scrambled egg whites, and 4 tablespoons cheese.
2 "always" carbohydrates, 2 "thumbs-up" proteins

Midmorning snack
Have 2 tablespoons peanuts with the apricots.
1 fruit, 1 "friendly" fat

Lunch
Add ¼ cup mashed avocado, ½ cup sliced bell peppers, and ½ cup sliced carrots to the spinach salad.

1 "always" carbohydrate, 1 "thumbs-up" protein, 1 "friendly" fat, 5 vegetables

TODAY'S TOTALS: 1,560 calories; 6 carbohydrates, 6 proteins, 2 fats, 2 fruits, 7+ vegetables

Day 3, Level 16

The same menu as Day 3, Level 12, except:

Midmorning snack	Have 2 tablespoons mixed nuts with the Cheerios. **1 "always" carbohydrate, 1 "friendly" fat**
Lunch	Have 1 large whole wheat pita pocket. **2 "always" carbohydrates, 1 "thumbs-up" protein, 2 vegetables**
Midafternoon snack	Have 2 tablespoons sunflower seeds with the yogurt. **1 fruit, 1 "thumbs-up" protein, 1 "friendly" fat**
Dinner	Have 4 ounces extra-lean ground beef with the pasta sauce. **2 "always" carbohydrates, 3 vegetables, 2 "thumbs-up" proteins**

**TODAY'S TOTALS: 1,608 calories; 6 carbohydrates, 6 proteins,
2 fats, 2 fruits, 5+ vegetables**

Day 4, Level 16

The same menu as Day 4, Level 12, except:

Breakfast	Have 1 cup oatmeal and ³/₄ cup cottage cheese. **2 "always" carbohydrates, 1¹/₂ "thumbs-up" proteins**
Midmorning snack	Have 1 flat tablespoon peanut butter. **¹/₂ fruit, 1 "friendly" fat**
Dinner	Add 1 teaspoon sesame oil and 1 tablespoon sesame seeds to the stir-fry. **2 "always" carbohydrates, 3 vegetables, 1¹/₂ "thumbs-up" proteins, 1 "friendly" fat**
After-dinner snack	Have 1 cup yogurt with the peach. **1 fruit, 1 "thumbs-up" protein**

**TODAY'S TOTALS: 1,575 calories; 6 carbohydrates, 6 proteins,
2 fruits, 2 fats, 5+ vegetables**

Day 5, Level 16

The same menu as Day 5, Level 12, except:

Breakfast Add 2 tablespoons pecan halves to the French toast topping.

1 "always" carbohydrate, 1 "thumbs-up" protein, 1 "friendly" fat

Lunch Have 4 ounces tuna on the sandwich.

2 "always" carbohydrates, 2 "thumbs-up" proteins, 2½ vegetables

Dinner Eat 1¼ cups brown rice or quinoa.

1½ "thumbs-up" proteins, 2½ "always" carbohydrates, 2 vegetables

After-dinner snack Have 2 tablespoons walnuts with the raisins.

1 fruit, 1 "friendly" fat

TODAY'S TOTALS: 1,569 calories; 6 carbohydrates, 6 proteins, 2 fruits, 2 fats, 4½+ vegetables

Day 6, Level 16

The same menu as Day 6, Level 12, except:

Breakfast Have 2 pancakes and 4 tablespoons sugar-free syrup or 2 tablespoons light syrup.

2 "always" carbohydrates, 1 fruit, 1 "thumbs-up" protein

Midmorning snack Put 1 tablespoon peanut butter in the celery stalk.

1 "friendly fat," ½ vegetable

Dinner Have 5 ounces of chicken.

1 "always" carbohydrate, 2½ "thumbs-up" proteins, 2 vegetables

After-dinner snack Top the baked apple with 2 tablespoons sliced pecans.

1 "friendly" fat, 1 fruit

TODAY'S TOTALS: 1,590 calories; 6 carbohydrates, 6 proteins, 2 fruits, 2 fats, 5½+ vegetables

Day 7, Level 16

The same menu as Day 7, Level 12, except:

Breakfast Have 2 slices whole wheat toast.
2 "always" carbohydrates, 1½ "thumbs-up" proteins, 1 vegetable

Midmorning snack Have 2 tablespoons pumpkin seeds with the watermelon.
1 fruit, 1 "friendly" fat

Lunch Have ¾ cup spiced chili beans and 1 ounce nonfat cheese on the potato.
1½ "always" carbohydrates, 2½ "thumbs-up" proteins, 2 vegetables

Midafternoon snack Add 2 teaspoons olive oil to the chickpea salad.
1 "always" carbohydrate, 1 vegetable, 1 "friendly" fat

TODAY'S TOTALS: 1,571 calories; 6 carbohydrates, 6 proteins, 2 fats, 2 fruits, 7+ vegetables

Day 8, Level 16

The same menu as Day 8, Level 12, except:

Midmorning snack Have the granola with the parfait.
1 "always" carbohydrate, 1 "sometimes" carbohydrate, 1 "thumbs-up" protein, 1 fruit

Lunch Have 4 ounces turkey breast on the English muffin.
2 "always" carbohydrates, 2 "thumbs-up" proteins, 2 vegetables

Midafternoon snack Have 1 tablespoon cashew butter.
1 "friendly" fat, 1 vegetable

After-dinner snack Add 2 tablespoons of slivered almonds to the raspberries.
1 fruit, 1 fat

TODAY'S TOTALS: 1,572 calories; 6 carbohydrates (5 "always," 1 "sometimes"), 6 proteins, 2 fruits, 2 fats, 5+ vegetables

Day 9, Level 16

The same menu as Day 9, Level 12, except:

Breakfast	Top waffle with 1 cup yogurt and add 2 tablespoons slivered pecans to the topping. **1 "always" carbohydrate, 1 "thumbs-up" protein, 1 "friendly" fat**
Midmorning snack	Have ½ cup cottage cheese. **1 fruit, 1 "thumbs-up" protein**
Lunch	Use 1 pita pocket. **2 "always" carbohydrates, 1 "thumbs-up" protein, ½ fruit, 2 vegetables**
Dinner	Use 4 tablespoons garlic sauce. **2 "always" carbohydrates, 2 "thumbs-up" proteins, 1 "friendly" fat, 4 vegetables**

TODAY'S TOTALS: 1,592 calories; 6 carbohydrates, 6 proteins, 2 fats, 2 fruits, 6+ vegetables

Day 10, Level 16

The same menu as Day 10, Level 12, except:

Midmorning snack	Make 4½ cups popcorn. **1½ "always" carbohydrates, 1 "thumbs-up" protein**
Lunch	Use the almond packet on the chicken salad (still hold the noodles). **2 "thumbs-up" proteins, 1 fruit, 2 "friendly" fats, 1½ vegetables**
Midafternoon snack	Have 1 small baked potato. **1 "always" carbohydrate, ½ "thumbs-up" protein, 1 vegetable**
Dinner	Use ½ cup egg substitute and 1 ounce cheese. **1 "always" carbohydrate, 2 "thumbs-up" proteins, 2½ vegetables**

TODAY'S TOTALS: 1,536 calories; 6 carbohydrates (5 "always," 1 "sometimes"), 6 proteins, 2 fats, 2 fruits, 5+ vegetables

Day 11, Level 16

The same menu as Day 11, Level 12, except:

Lunch	Use 1 whole-grain bun for the mushroom burger. Add 2 tablespoons slivered almonds to the strawberry salad.
	2 "always" carbohydrates, ³/₄ "thumbs-up" protein, 1 fruit, 1 fat, 2¹/₂ vegetables
Midafternoon snack	Add 2 flat tablespoons light mayo to ¹/₂ sandwich (or use mustard or ketchup on the sandwich and add 4 tablespoons almonds to the salad at lunch).
	1 "sometimes" carbohydrate, 1 fat "foe," 1 "thumbs-up" protein, ¹/₂ vegetable
Dinner	Have 5 ounces salmon.
	1 "always" carbohydrate, 2³/₄ "thumbs-up" proteins, 2 vegetables

TODAY'S TOTALS: 1,575 calories; 6 carbohydrates (5 "always," 1 "sometimes"), 6 "thumbs-up" proteins, 2 fats (1 "friendly," 1 "foe"), 2 fruits, 5+ vegetables

Day 12, Level 16

The same menu as Day 12, Level 12, except:

Breakfast	Use 2 slices bread for the French toast. Also use 4 egg whites (or ¹/₂ cup fat-free egg substitute).
	2 "always" carbohydrates, 1 "thumbs-up" protein
Midmorning snack	Cut the apple in quarters so that you can spread 1 flat tablespoon peanut butter on top of the apple pieces.
	1 fruit, 1 "thumbs-up" protein, 1 "friendly" fat
Dinner	Use 4¹/₂ ounces extra-lean beef in the stir-fry.
	2 "always" carbohydrates, 2¹/₄ "thumbs-up" proteins, ¹/₂ "friendly" fat, 4¹/₂ vegetables
After-dinner snack	Mix 1 tablespoon sunflower seeds into the yogurt.
	¹/₂ "always" carbohydrate, 1 fruit, ¹/₂ fat

TODAY'S TOTALS: 1,605 calories; 6 carbohydrates, 6 proteins, 2 fruits, 2 fats, 6¹/₂+ vegetables

Day 13, Level 16

The same menu as Day 13, Level 12, except:

Breakfast   Also eat 1 slice whole wheat toast.

1³/₄ "always" carbohydrates, ¹/₄ "thumbs-up" protein, 1 fruit

Midmorning snack   Add 2 tablespoons slivered almonds or another nut of your choice to the bananas and cream.

1 "thumbs-up" protein, 1 fruit, 1 "friendly" fat

Lunch   Have 4 ounces crabmeat. Add 1 ounce (about 4 small cubes) avocado to the watercress and cucumber salad.

¹/₂ "always" carbohydrate, 2 "thumbs-up" proteins, ¹/₂ "friendly" fat, 2¹/₂ vegetables

---

TODAY'S TOTALS: 1,540 calories; 6 carbohydrates (5 "always," 1 "rarely"), 6 proteins, 2 fruits, 2 fats, 6¹/₂+ vegetables

Day 14, Level 16

The same menu as Day 14, Level 12, except:

Midmorning snack   Spread 1¹/₄ tablespoons peanut butter (instead of spray) on the bread.

¹/₂ "always" carbohydrate, ¹/₂ "thumbs-up" protein, 1¹/₄ "friendly" fats

Lunch   Use 2 ounces tuna and 1 ounce cheese. Eat the same size salad or more.

1 "always" carbohydrate, 2 "thumbs-up" proteins, 2¹/₂ vegetables

Midafternoon snack   Have ¹/₄ cup Grape-Nuts.

1 "always" carbohydrate, ¹/₂ "thumbs-up" protein, 1 fruit

TODAY'S TOTALS: 1,551 calories; 6 carbohydrates, 6 proteins, 2 fruits, 2 fats, 4³/₄+ vegetables

INDEX

beef, ground, 85, 86, 92–93
Beef stir-fry, 286
bench press, 251
berries, 72
biceps curls, 247, 253
bisque, 110
blood sugar, 57–58, 60, 83, 106
blueberries, 72
body fat percentage, 48–49, 236 *see also* fat, body
body needs, computing, 63–66
brain, fuel for, 200
bran, 58, 59
breads
  in "always" carbohydrate group, 23
  before meals, 75
  choosing, 61
  myth buster, 45
  snack/mini-meals, 168–69
  in "sometimes" carbohydrate group, 27
  in ten-day breakfast cycle, 142, 143, 145, 148
  whole-grain, 26, 60
breakfast, 128–51
  carbohydrates for, 137–39
  choosing food for, 136, 139–40
  effects of skipping, 133–34
  fruit for, 140
  fuel provided in, 131, 135
  importance of, 129
  myth busters, 128–29
  nausea from, 141–42
  starting slowly from zero with, 135, 141
  ten-day cycle, 142–51
  tips about, 132–33, 134–35, 136–37, 138, 139, 140
  twin trial, 129–31
  and weight loss, 131–32
breakfast bars, 134
breathing, deep, 205
bridge mix, 162

broccoli, 68
bubble baths, 201–2, 209
buffalo meat, 88
bungee tubing, 246, 247, 248, 257
butter, 40
butt, exercises for, 244, 249, 255, 257

caffeine, 135, 183–84, 186, 206
calcium, 99
calcium supplement, 203
calories
  burning of, 16, 17, 19, 49, 60, 83, 131, 138, 151, 164, 199, 211–12
  divided among extra meals, 164–68
  and exercise, 208, 211–12
  and metabolism, 1, 17
CamelBak, 189
canned foods
  exercising with, 257
  sodium in, 69
cantaloupe, 132, 156
carbohydrates, 19–31, 44–76
  "always," 20, 21–26
  bad, 57–63
  for breakfast, 137–39
  and burning body fat, 51–52
  cravings for, 203, 204–5
  daily servings of, 65–66, 89
  and fats, 38, 52–53, 109, 112, 114–15
  fiber in, 20, 59, 60, 138–39
  as fuel, 49, 160, 200
  functions of, 17, 19
  how to eat, 52–57
  and muscle, 49, 50, 160, 200
  myth busters, 44–45
  portions of, 22, 54–57, 62
  and protein, 31, 32, 38, 83
  "rarely," 20–21, 29–31
  and sleep, 200, 204–5
  snack/mini-meals, 168–71
  "sometimes," 20–21, 26–29
  sources of, 17

cross-training, 214, 228
crunch exercise, 248, 254
curb-ups, 249

dairy products, 32, 99–101
  low-fat and nonfat, 78, 118, 123
  milk on cereal, 75
  snack/mini-meals, 172
  as "thumbs-down" protein, 36–37
  as "thumbs-up" protein, 33–35
  tips about, 100–101
  warm skim milk, 162
dancing, 213, 218
deep-breathing technique, 205
dehydration, 181–82, 190–91, 192
delta sleep, 202
deprivation, feelings of, 30
diary, food, 13–14, 41, 42–43
diet-induced thermogenesis, 60, 131,
    133, 134, 137, 138–39, 159, 164
dieting
  and carbohydrates, 50, 51, 52
  chronic, 2
  deprivation feelings from, 30
  and metabolism, 2, 16
  semistarvation, 107
  and stomach capacity, 162
  water loss in, 50, 51
dog at hydrant exercise, 250
doggie bags, 165
dog walking, 220
drowsiness, 199
dumbbell exercise, 252
dumbbell flye, 251
dumbbell kick back, 247
dumbbell press, 253
dust, 200–201

earplugs, 205
eating out, doggie bags from, 165
eccentric phase, 257
edamame, 97, 158
eggs, 101
  and cholesterol, 128–29

cooking spray used with, 137, 140
omelets, 137
scrambled, 140, 156
as "thumbs-up" protein, 33
electrolytes, 190
endorphins, 211, 214
endosperm, 57, 58
energy
  burning calories via, 17, 19
  burning fat stores for, 108–9
  carbohydrates as fuel for, 49
  from fats, 105, 106
  protein as alternative fuel for, 49,
    51, 87
  and sugar, 21, 29, 71
  temporary, 57
  and water, 181, 182
energy bars, 74
English muffin pizza, 270
exercise, 207–28
  appointment for, 224
  benefits of, 211, 222
  building muscle with, see exercises
  and calories, 208, 211–12
  cardiovascular, 212, 213–14, 217
  clothing and gear for, 212, 214, 217
  commitment to, 223, 224
  cross-training, 214, 228
  digestion time before, 260
  excuses vs., 214, 221
  fuel for, 160
  goals for, 222
  as habit, 226–28
  imagery in, 225–26
  intensity of, 215–17
  interval training, 226–27
  MAGIC for, 222–26
  motivation for, 222–24
  myth busters, 207–8
  personal trainer for, 224, 236–37
  plateauing in, 207
  positive affirmations in, 225–26
  rewards for, 226
  and sleep, 202

push down the wall, 243, 246
push-up, 245–46

quadriceps, exercises for, 244
  horizontal leg press, 255
  leg extension, 255
  stair walking, 250
quiche, 126–27

radial pulse, 217
raise on tiptoes exercise, 250
raisin bran, 59–60, 139
Raisin French toast, 285
raisins, 72
reaching, 220
recipes
  Banana smoothie, 133
  Barley and bean salad, 289
  Beef stir-fry, 286
  Chinese take-out, 278
  Crab-stuffed tomato, 288
  Crispy oven-fried fired-up chicken,
    289–90
  English muffin pizza, 270
  French toast, 268
  Grilled cheese pita sandwich, 277
  Mexican chicken wrap, 260–61
  Mexican fajita, 276
  Open-faced egg and cheese muffin,
    262
  Open-faced portobello mushroom
    burger, 282
  Orange chicken, 271
  Oven-fried potatoes, 54
  Peachy smoothie, 288
  Potato chips, 113
  Raisin French toast, 285
  Rosemary chicken, 274
  Salmon and dill, 283
  Shrimp or tofu stir-fry, 267
  Spaghetti with meat and vegetable
    sauce, 265
  Spicy egg burrito, 280
  Spinach salad, 262

Strawberry salad, 282
Tomato artichoke salad, 291–92
Tuna melt, 291
Tuna sandwich, 268
Turkey sandwich, 266
Veggie melt, 264
Yogurt parfait, 279
refrigerator, clearing out, 164
relaxation, 163, 202, 205
resistance ball, 220
restaurant, doggie bags from,
  165
reverse crunch, 248, 254
reward, 226
rice
  and beans, 158
  brown, 62
  "bulking up" as it cooks, 12
rice cakes, 75
Rosemary chicken, 274
rotation trunk curl, 254–55
Rule of Hand, 12–13, 33
  for grains, 62–63
  for protein, 92
running, 207

salad, 69, 101, 105
salad dressings/sandwich spreads
  in fat "foes" group, 40–41
  in "friendly" fats group, 39–40
  in snack/mini-meals, 175
  substitutes, 123
salmon, smoked (lox), 132
Salmon and dill, 283
San Pellegrino, 190
saturated fat, 93, 110
sausage, 115
scallops, 93
scapular adduction, 252
seafood, see fish
seeds, see nuts and seeds
self-control, 14–15, 16
seltzer, 185, 190
serotonin, 205

sheets, cotton, 204
shoes, comfortable, 221
shoulders, exercises for
   bungee tubing, 246, 257
   dumbbell press, 253
   lateral shoulder raise, 253
   push-up, 245–46
   scapular adduction, 252
   shoulder press, 247
   tips about, 257
shoveling, 221
shower, warm, 201–2
shrimp, 95
Shrimp or tofu stir-fry, 267
side shuffle, 250, 258
skim latte, 136
skipping, 215
skipping breakfast, *see* breakfast
skipping meals, 152–76
   adding extra meals, 164–65
   benefits of eating frequently, 155, 156
   fuel for exercise, 160
   hindering habits, 166–68
   myth busters, 152–53
   and shrinking stomach, 161–62
   and slowing metabolism, 159–60
   small, frequent meals vs., 159–60, 162
   snack/mini-meal lists, 168–76
   snacks, 162–64
   spreading out lunch, 165–68
   tips, 155–56, 157–58, 160–61, 162, 163–64
   twin trial, 153–55
sleep, 194–206
   appointment for, 200
   body in conservation mode, 129
   body requirement of, 198
   and carbohydrates, 200, 204–5
   delta, 202
   deprivation, 198–200, 203
   and hunger, 199, 203–5

   myth busters, 194–95
   and noise, 198, 205
   with pets, 206
   and serotonin, 205
   tips about, 198, 200–206
   twin trial, 195–97
smoothies, 133, 134, 157, 288
snacks
   after-dinner, 32
   before bedtime, 200
   benefits of, 161–62
   carbohydrates for, 168–71
   drinking water before, 182–83
   fats for, 174–75
   healthful alternatives, 175–76
   midmorning, 155–56
   as mini-meals, 162–63
   pre-exercise, 160
   proteins for, 172–73
   soups, 156, 158, 171, 175
   and spreading out lunch, 166–68
   timing of, 164
   tips for, 156, 157–58, 160–61, 162, 163–64
   and weight gain, 164–65
   and weight loss, 156, 160
sneezing, 219
soda, 59, 184, 185, 186, 192
sodium
   in canned foods, 69
   diluting, 188
sole, fillet of, 96
soup
   for breakfast, 140
   for snacks, 156, 158, 171, 175
soy nuts, 106
soy products, 96–97
   "friendly" fats and, 105
   in snack/mini-meals, 173, 176
   see also tofu
Spaghetti with meat and vegetable sauce, 265
Special K, 56, 57
Spicy egg burrito, 280

yoga, 217
yogurt, 100–101
    in "always" carbohydrate group,
      26
    benefits of, 32
    full-fat, 136
    in "rarely" carbohydrate group, 31

    in smoothies, 134
    in snacks, 156
    stir-in, 140
    in ten-day breakfast cycle, 143, 145
    as "thumbs-down" protein, 37
    as "thumbs-up" protein, 35
Yogurt parfait, 279

ABOUT THE AUTHORS

Right down to their refrigerators, which are stuffed with matching items, LYSSIE LAKATOS and TAMMY LAKATOS SHAMES are identical twins. Registered dietitians, they founded Healthy Happenings, a company that counsels individuals and has provided nutrition seminars for corporations including AOL Time Warner, Colgate-Palmolive, Standard and Poor's, UAW-Ford Motor, and *The New York Times*. Lyssie and Tammy's clients also include celebrities, professional athletes, the U.S. Eco-Challenge team, the top players on the Worldwide Senior Tennis Circuit, and participants in varied races and marathons.

The Lakatos sisters appear regularly as nutrition experts on The Discovery Health Channel, and they have contributed to print and online publications including *Self*, *Good Housekeeping*, *Woman's Day*, *Health*, *Parents*, *Woman's World*, *First for Women*, and *Family Circle;* as well as the WebMD, Weight Watchers, and Fit to Be Tied websites.

They live in New York City.